# INFORMATION MANAGEMENT IN HEALTH CARE

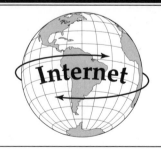

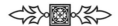

# INFORMATION
# MANAGEMENT
# IN HEALTH CARE

**Richard D. Marreel, BS, CDP**
President, R. Marreel & Associates
Colorado Springs, Colorado

**Janet M. McLellan, RN MSN, CNA**
President, The McLellan Group, Inc.
Colorado Springs, Colorado
Assistant Department Chair, Nursing, Colorado
University of Phoenix

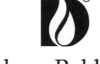
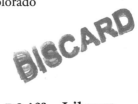

## Delmar Publishers

*an International Thomson Publishing company*

Albany • Bonn • Boston • Cincinnati • Detroit • London • Madrid
Melbourne • Mexico City • New York • Pacific Grove • Paris • San Francisco
Singapore • Tokyo • Toronto • Washington

# NOTICE TO THE READER

Cover Design:   *Timothy J. Conners*

**Delmar Staff**
Publisher:   *William Brottmiller*
Acquisitions Editor:   *Marion Waldman*
Editorial Assistant:   *Diane Biondi*
Production Coordinator:   *Sandra Woods*
Art/Design Coordinator:   *Timothy J. Conners*

COPYRIGHT © 1999
By Delmar Publishers, Inc.
an International Thomson Publishing Company

The ITP logo is a trademark under license.

Printed in the United States of America

For more information, contact:

Delmar Publishers, Inc.
3 Columbia Circle, Box 15015
Albany, New York 12212-5015

International Thomson Publishing
Berkshire House
168-173 High Holborn
London, WC1V7AA
United Kingdom

Nelson ITP, Australia
102 Dodds Street
South Melbourne 3205
Victoria, 3205 Australia

Nelson Canada
1120 Birchmont Road
Scarborough, Ontario
M1K 5G4, Canada

International Thomson Publishing France
Tour Maine-Montparnasse
33 Avenue du Maine
75755 Paris Cedex 15, France

International Thomson Editores
Seneca 53
Colonia Polanco
11560 Mexico D F Mexico

International Thomson Publishing GmbH
Königswinterer Stasße. 418
53227 Bonn
Germany

International Thomson Publishing Asia
60 Albert Street
#15-01 Albert Complex
Singapore 189969

International Thomson Publishing Japan
Hirakawa-cho Kyowa Building, 3F
2-2-1 Hirakawa-cho, Chiyoda-ku,
Tokyo 102, Japan

ITE Spain Paraninfo
Calle Magallanes, 25
28015-Madrid, Espana

1 2 3 4 5 6 7 8 9 10 XXX 03 02 01 00 99 98

**Library of Congress Cataloging-in-Publication Data**

Marreel, Richard D.
    Information management in health care / Richard D. Marreel, Janet
M. McLellan
        p.   cm.
    Includes bibliographical references and index.
    ISBN 0-7668-1255-3
    1. Medicine—Data processing.   2. Information storage and
retrieval systems—Medical care.   3. Information resources
management.   I. McLellan, Janet M.   II. Title.
R858.M375 1999
610'.285—dc21                                      98-51743
                                               CIP

# CONTENTS

# PREFACE

Computer automation is pervasive in today's society. Everywhere we turn automation is in evidence. The grocery store has automated scanners and even automated checkout lines. The bank has automated tellers, check scanners, and wire transfers. The library has automated catalogs and interlibrary lending. From our homes, we can access the world through the Internet, and purchase just about anything, from shares of Microsoft to Sunday's dinner, through our personal computers. A litany of computerized marvels could fill volumes.

The explosion of new technology over the past twenty years that makes all of this possible is truly phenomenal. What is even more phenomenal, and perhaps a little frightening, is that this is just the beginning. The time will come, in the not too distant future, when the thoughts, communications, creations, manuscripts, learning material, and financial assets of the civilized world will exist primarily in electronic form. If the lights went out, civilization as we know it would cease to exist.

Health care is not immune. Some of the most complex systems, and certainly some of the most complex system requirements, can be found in the field of health care. Systems to serve the diverse needs of administration, patient management, finance, materials management, billing and collections, decision support, managed care, nursing, operating room, emergency room, clinics, laboratory, imaging, intensive care, pharmacy, telemedicine, long-term care, home care, and physicians' offices need to be implemented and integrated across the continuum of care of modern health care provider organizations. As a result, the demand for health care professionals who are knowledgeable in the application of technology is growing rapidly.

Even with technology all around us, we do not always feel comfortable with it. Technology is sometimes confusing, intimidating, and in large part because it changes so rapidly, downright bewildering. In spite of the continual changes, some relative constants make the field less confusing and easier to manage. One of the biggest challenges we face is how to properly harness and apply the available technology. The good news is that while the technology will continue to change, the techniques employed to apply the technology do not. The purpose of this book is to convey and demonstrate the application of these techniques in the health care setting.

Anyone involved in health care delivery can benefit from the concepts, methodologies, and techniques discussed in this book. It is of particular value to health care administrators, chief information officers, and staff involved in information management planning and/or the selection, implementation, and support of automated systems.

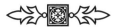

# CHAPTER

## 1

# Introduction

Let us start at the beginning. The computer age began in the mid 1800s. Some historians argue that the abacus was the first rudimentary calculating tool. For our discussion, we will look at the first mechanical calculating machine. Charles Babbage, in 1834, designed the "analytical engine" that was a general all-purpose calculating machine, controlled by a sequence of instructions. This steam-powered device contained a processing unit, a main storage area, input and output data, and step-by-step control (Hyman, 1982). One observer wrote, "the Analytical Engine has no pretensions whatever to originate anything. It can do whatever we know how to order it to perform" (Bowden, 1953). There were very few prototypes made of the analytical engine, and the ideas and design lay dormant for almost a century.

In the 1930s and 1940s, there was an intense effort to develop a digital electronic computer. In 1936, Alan Turing proposed a computer design that could, in theory, solve any problem that could be stated in the form of an algorithm. In 1946, John Van Neumann designed a computer controlled by a stored program. The machine was to operate on data and instructions in a binary code stored together in memory (Bishop, 1986).

As these prototypes continued to prove successful, the first commercial electronic computer was produced as the "Univac" in 1951. These early models ran on valves and were very large and clumsy. In other research, the transistor had been invented in 1948, and computers as we know them today became a reality. Transistors were small, cheap, and very reliable. Several were placed on a single integrated circuit board, which has became known as "the chip." In the 1960s, International Business Machines (IBM) had the first commercial series of computers on the market. The late 1960s and the early 1970s saw the first health care computing systems used primarily for registration and billing.

It was not until the 1970s that health care information systems were implemented. In 1973, the Technicon Medical Information System was developed and implemented at El Camino Hospital in Mountain View, California, by Lockheed Corporation. This early edition managed all patient information during the hospital stay. It consisted of nursing care protocols generated from patients' medical diagnoses and predicted outcome measures that were used as guidelines to record patient problems and care plans. This system ran on a mainframe computer that supported a large number of "dumb terminals," activated by a light pen (Cook & Mayers, 1981).

From that first implementation, there have been hundreds of hospitals that have implemented the Technicon system. While the ownership of the company has changed hands several times, after thirty years, it is still one of the most advanced health information systems (HISs). Recently, this system has undergone a major overhaul, and its hardware architecture and software have been upgraded to operate in a client-server environment with industry standard hardware and software components.

Computers, like all tools, were developed and refined to make tasks easier and faster. The first computers performed specific tasks and were not easily modified. They could be compared to a music box. Once wound up, they played the same tune over and over again. A music box is both reliable and consistent. There are no missed notes, and the tempo is always the same. Originally mechanical computers were much the same, performing calculations on numeric data entered into the computer in a rigorously applied format, producing sums, averages, products, and quotients time after time, with great consistency and reliability. The benefit of these early machines was their ability to produce these results quickly and accurately by removing the variability introduced through human error. The computer freed human operators from the repetitive calculation tasks, so they could concentrate on acquisition of good data, thereby improving both productivity and quality.

## HARDWARE

The computer consists of four interacting components: the central processing unit, the input devices and output devices, and storage components (see Figure 1–1). We call these components *hardware.* We will look at each component briefly.

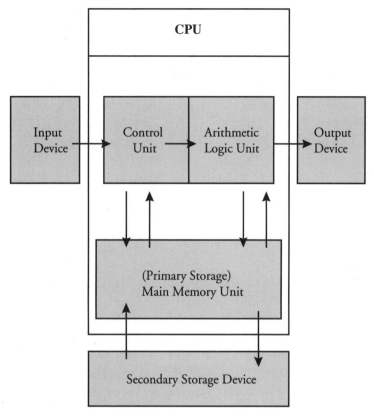

**Figure 1–1** Four functional components of the computer (Saba & McCormick, 1996)

## Central Processing Unit (CPU)

The CPU has two parts, the control, or processing, unit and the arithmetic logic unit. The control unit reads the program instructions, determines the sequence of events, and routes the data to different parts of the computer. The actual comparison of data or the activities of addition and subtraction are done in the logic unit.

## Input and Output Devices

In order for the users to communicate with the computer, there must be input and output devices. Common input and output devices used are keyboards, monitors, and printers. The monitor consists of a glass screen, somewhat like a television screen, where information can be displayed. Attached to the screen, is a keyboard for typing or keying information into the computer. There are several types and styles of keyboards. New models are combining ergonomically correct features like splitting the hand placement and raising the wrists and forearms into more neutral positions. There are even models that feature different placement of the letters and numbers. Some health care systems use light pens, probe pens, touch screens, bar code readers, and voice activation, as well as the keyboard, as input devices. Many of these have proven faster and more accurate than typing information onto the screen.

Once the data is in the computer, it is manipulated into information and is stored until it is needed. The output device, usually a printer, is used to print selected information. Printed output or material is called "hard copy." Printers come in all sizes, qualities and speeds of printing. There are ink-jet, daisy wheel, dot matrix, and laser printers, as well as color and black-only printers. The user must identify the specific use for each printer to ensure the right combination is being purchased.

## Storage Devices

Each computer needs a place to store data and information before and after it is processed. The main memory or microchip is built into the computer. As the microchip has increased in capacity, main memory also has increased. The main memory has limited space and can be quickly used up with the immense software programs that are being produced today.

The computer uses permanent magnetic disks, floppy disks, compact discs (CDs), and magnetic tapes for secondary storage. Permanent magnetic disks can be quite large in capacity and provide the fastest access to data on computers in common use. Floppy disks are small, only three and one-half inches, but can store between 720 kilobytes (KB) and 1.44 megabytes (MB) of information. A CD provides greater storage density but is relatively slow when it comes to storage and retrieval of data. Tapes come in three sizes: (1) the cassette, similar to an audiocassette; (2) the cartridge, used for backup purposes, and (3) the much larger reel-to-reel tape. Tape storage is used primarily for backing up current data, from permanent magnetic disk, for recovery in case of loss, and for archival of inactive data.

## SOFTWARE

The next step in the evolution of the computer was the introduction of the concept of software. Through this innovation, the same computer could be given instructions to perform different tasks. We can compare this next stage of evolution to a player piano. Like the music box, we are still producing music, but now the music can be changed, depending on the instructions provided to the piano. The player piano represents the two basic components of modern computers—the instrument that produces the music (hardware), and the roll of paper with punched holes that instructs the piano which tune is to be played (software).

## Operating System

Initially, due to the limitations of available technology, the computer user had to be satisfied with loading each software program on the computer individually, much the same as changing a song roll on the player piano. As technology improved, specialized software programs were developed to enable the computer to manage its own work. With this new software, computers could perform several different tasks at the same time—calculating, accepting new data from outside sources, storing data, displaying information, and so on. This specialized software is referred to as the operating system.

Thus, we have completed a description of the three basic layers involved in computing: the hardware, the application software, and the operating system software. In spite of all the improvements to the technology and the techniques used to build these three components, they will remain basic to computers into the foreseeable future. Computers large and small, costing less than a thousand dollars or several million dollars, all have these components in common. They differ only in speed, complexity, and capabilities.

Unless you are a computer programmer or software engineer, you will be most concerned with application software. These are the programs that "play the music." Our concern through the rest of this book is to describe the tools and methodologies that will enable you to select and implement application software products that are harmonious with the current and future needs of your health care organization.

## Application Software

Application software is developed to meet the specific needs of an organization or industry sector. In the health care sector, applications have been developed primarily to meet the needs of administration, finance, and patient care. In the early 1970s, large health care organizations hired programmers and analysts to develop software, but this proved to be very expensive and time-consuming. The health care industry found itself changing faster than new software could be developed or old software could be modified. Consequently, self-developed software became impractical for all but the very largest health care organizations.

Most application software used today is acquired from software vendors able to spread their development and modification costs over a large group of customers. While initial acquisition costs can still be quite high, sometimes several million dollars, ongoing maintenance and improvement costs are much more manageable and predictable.

## OVERALL SYSTEM CHARACTERISTICS

How should these software packages be designed? There are generally accepted system characteristics that all health care organizations are looking for, just by the nature of their business needs (Zielstorff, McHugh, & Clinton, 1988). Consider each of the elements discussed in the following text when selecting a new software system or assessing an old system.

## Flexibility

The software application must have the ability to be configured at the health care site to meet the model of care the organization currently uses. Organization-specific items like vocabulary, decision rules, standing orders, reports, and displays should be configured as is and not have to be changed. Changes should be made only at the option of the organization.

The software application must be upgradeable. That is to say, as the industry improves the product, your current software should have the capability to be upgraded. These improvements should apply to all the existing data on the system. The system also should be adaptable to the changing data reporting requirements of external agencies and new methods of delivering care.

## Connectivity

To avoid duplication of work, the application software should communicate with all other software in the health care organization. The application software should support standard communication protocols to enable data sharing.

Communication links to external software applications, such as data banks or bibliographic retrievals and other media resources, are necessary. The software application should be able to contribute to external databases, as well as retrieve data from other software systems.

## Performance

The application software should provide continuous service. With the health care organization being a twenty-four-hour service, the software system cannot be down for backups.

Testing at peak times of use should demonstrate satisfactory performance for all software applications.

## Security and Confidentiality

Reliability and integrity of data should be assured, so data can be captured, transmitted, stored, and displayed without error. Security codes and unique user identification should be protected and generated automatically. Audit trails should be kept on all transactions. If errors are made, they should be flagged as such, not deleted.

Confidentiality of data should be maintained. Screen savers, timed sign-ons and sign-offs, and complex algorithms that encrypt unique patient and provider identifiers should be used before data is sent to national or state agencies for research and inquiry.

## Human Factors

The software application and hardware components must accommodate a variety of input methods. Data capturing must be less time-consuming than manual methods, whenever possible. Comfortable vocabulary must be used.

The software application should follow logical work flow. It should be intuitive about what comes next. Pathways should be easily followed.

Connectivity to other software applications, either internal or external, should be seamless. Due to the difficulties inherent in the connecting of legacy or existing systems with new systems, this might be impossible, but it should be a goal of the organization.

## COMMON SOFTWARE APPLICATIONS

Although not all of the health care software lends itself to a tidy classification, the following applications are commonly found in health care organizations throughout the country:

**Administrative**
- Executive decision support
- Patient management
- Medical staff credentialing
- Materials management
- Managed care
- Human resources/benefits management
- Staff scheduling
- Operating room (OR) scheduling
- E-mail

**Financial**
- Patient accounting
- Accounts receivable management
- Cost accounting
- Accounts payable

- General accounting
- Payroll

**Patient Care**
- HIS
  — Order entry/results reporting
  — Charting
  — Care planning
- Patient education
- Laboratory
- Radiology
- Physician practice management
- Pharmacy
- Telemedicine
- Home care
- Patient scheduling
- Patient acuity

These applications are available from a variety of different vendors and are installed on many different hardware and operating system configurations. The hardware, or the machine that runs an application, is referred to as the "hardware platform." The operating system that runs the application software is called the "system platform."

Hardware vendors, such as International Business Machines (IBM), Hewlett Packard (HP), or Digital Equipment Corporation (DEC), provide several different hardware and system platforms, depending upon the needs of the application vendor. Application vendors in turn can offer several application alternatives depending on the needs of their customers.

As a result, there can be considerable variation among health care organizations in regard to how each accomplishes a similar automation task. Patient registration, for example, could be automated as a single function on a microcomputer, commonly referred to as a personal computer (PC), or on a midrange computer, otherwise known as a minicomputer, or on a large computer, known as a mainframe. The patient registration application can operate all by itself (stand alone), as a part of a larger network of software applications (client-server network), or as an integrated part of a complete HIS located on a mainframe.

It is because of this variation in needs and expectations from automation that the job of selecting the "right" system can be very intimidating. Many issues need to be addressed: functionality, expandability, operating environment, degree of integration required, cost relative to expected benefits, maintenance and support requirements, required implementation and training effort, and compatibility with existing systems—to name just a few.

Using the tools presented and described in subsequent chapters, you will be able to sort out all these variables and make an informed decision on whether to automate, and if so, which products and services will best fit your needs.

## APPLICATION DESCRIPTIONS

### Executive Decision System (EDS) or Executive Information System (EIS)

An EDS can meet several needs of a health care administration. It provides the ability to:

- Explore—to create new perspectives, reports, and graphs
- Identify variance analysis—to contrast relationships between existing data and new information
- Propose "what if" analysis—to evaluate the impact of one change upon another
- Provide computer modeling—to manipulate the data and change the rules upon which the data is based
- Electronically generate reports—to provide easy access to existing information
- Customize reports—to modify existing reports, and to use color coding and drill down features

### Patient Management

As a patient enters an organization, a minimum data set of information must be collected. Patient management software applications assist with the collection and management of admission, discharge, and transfer information. A systematic approach is necessary to have access to the same information, about the same patient, everywhere in the system. Many times there is a separate patient management module within the HIS, but not always.

### Medical Staff Credentialing

Federal law requires that every health care organization maintain detailed records on physicians and health care extenders. Each health care entity has rules and regulations concerning educational requirements, certifications, codes of conduct, practice acts, and so on. Credentialing software applications make this process more efficient and provide the ability to generate reports for submission to local, state, and federal regulatory agencies.

## Materials Management

Not long ago, materials management application software was strictly inventory accounting and replenishment checklists. These applications have evolved into comprehensive information management tools. They offer more sophisticated features, ranging from electronic data interchange capability to bar code input devices. They provide information for decisions to be made at the lowest level, so decisions can be made at the point of contact, right in the patient's room (Darnell, 1996).

## Managed Care

Managed care software is usually comprised of modules specializing in patient eligibility checking, contract administration, contract modeling, financial risk management, health management organization (HMO) and physician provider organizaiton (PPO) administration, and workers' compensation issues. The massive swing to the managed care model of health care has brought intense focus on the needs of organizations dealing with these care contracts.

## Human Resources—Benefits Management

As health care organizations grow larger and more complex, software applications are invaluable for organizing information. Every employee has a data set that must be kept current and accurate. Human resource and benefits management software applications provide the ability to maintain employment-related data on employees, and design and manage any number of complex benefit packages.

## Staff Scheduling

Introduction to staff scheduling programs came in the 1980s. Many health care organizations joined the cause, only to find that scheduling systems fell short. Many organizations shelved their early staff scheduling products and have returned to manually generating schedules. When assessing a scheduling software package, evaluate the product against these outcomes:

- Optimum allocation of available staff resources to match staffing needs
- Equitable treatment of staff in their work schedules
- Accurate and timely information

Software applications containing these four elements will improve satisfaction of a staff scheduling system by:

- Minimizing personnel time in schedule creation
- Eliminating redundancy of data
- Maintaining authority and control with desired management levels
- Minimizing paper documents and manual data recording and flow

Successful scheduling depends on the existence of effective management systems, including full-time employee (FTE) and position control, proper request management, well-defined data and work flow, and timeline management (Hanson, 1993).

## Operating Room (OR) Scheduling

In today's health care organizations, the operating rooms produce high revenue and can be used for both inpatient and outpatient services. It is imperative that the process runs smoothly and efficiently. Operating room software applications specialize in scheduling rooms and equipment, estimating times for each type of surgery, and providing supply lists based on physician preference.

## E-mail

E-mail has gone from a convenience to a mission critical application. It is the backbone to collecting and distributing information and communications both within and outside an organization. Messages may be sent anytime, from any terminal, with the ability to tag a message for receipt upon being read. These software applications alert users when a message is sitting on the server, waiting for them to retrieve it. Some proprietary software applications include group scheduling and calendar management.

Policies and procedures should be reviewed with the implementation of an E-mail system. These software applications are not usually secure enough to send confidential data. With a single click of the mouse, one message can be sent to every workstation in an organization. Announcing a vacation trip over E-mail could be inviting a burglar to break into your home. Unless saved, E-mail messages are deleted immediately from the system. Knowledge of the capabilities of the system increases the acceptance and use.

## Financial Systems

Health care decision makers realize that in today's competitive, cost-conscious environment, they need to have good information to survive and compete. Maintaining control of the money that flows in and out of a health care organization can be overwhelming. Many have determined they must re-engineer their financial systems to better utilize information and reduce costs. It takes several software applications working in collaboration to give an accurate picture. Prominent among those are:

- Patient accounting
- Accounts payable
- Accounts receivable management
- General accounting
- Cost accounting
- Payroll

In addition to these basic systems, finance is looking for:

- Electronic data interchange (EDI)
- Internet and Intranet applications
- Year 2000 compliant software
- Data warehouses

Straub (1997) reported, "Currently systems are either very simplistic and easy-to-use, or complex and hard-to-use. We need Nirvana—systems that are powerful, easy-to-use and manipulate. Until then, the current systems will be under utilized."

## Electronic Data Interchange (EDI)—Claims and Purchasing

Federal legislation will assist the continued movement toward electronic claims submission. The Health Insurance Portability and Accountability Act contained a provision requiring most payers to be capable of handling claims and related transactions in standard electronic formats by the year 2000. Among payers, Medicare and Medicaid continue to lead the way toward automation. The Health Care Financing Administration (HCFA) is no longer focusing on getting more claims in electronically, but on standardizing electronic claims formats and the formats of other related transactions. This will assist in consistency and standardization across the industry (Goedert, 1996).

Many providers rely on EDI technology to improve their supply chain, as well as reduce the utilization of supplies. These providers are saving time and money by using technology such as the Internet, bar coding, purchasing cards (used just like credit cards), and automated supply stations (McCormack, 1997). By using patient-centered delivery methods, they are eliminating bulk storage and excessive departmental inventories. By capturing every charge and not having to store large quantities, health care organizations are saving millions.

## Health Information System (HIS)

Health information systems have been developing since the early 1970s. Vast improvements to existing modules and new modules are coming on the market every year. The goal for most health care organizations is to have an electronic patient record—no paper. The reality of this is several years off. There are so many separate functions within a health care organization, it is very difficult to have one vendor be "the best" at everything. Vendors have specialized in certain areas over the years, forcing many organizations to implement a hodgepodge of "best of breed" software applications. To get to the goal of an electronic patient record, all these disparate systems must talk to one another by passing patient data across all systems effortlessly and seamlessly to the user. Common modules found in a HIS are:

- **Order Entry and Results Reporting.** This is a series of pathways for entering an order into the system. It travels to the correct department or area, and it is scheduled, completed, and charged for within the system. Results reporting follows. When a result is documented into the system, it appears in the patient's file for review by all caregivers.
- **Charting.** Every caregiver must record any care activity, and the reaction to that care, on a patient chart. With an electronic medical record, the "chart" is on-line and available to everyone who has a need to know. Many HISs have a charting module. Implementing the module causes a shift in work patterns and requires education of the health care workers. The benefits outweigh the distress, by allowing access throughout the organization.
- **Care Planning.** Monitoring a patient's progress is difficult if there is not a plan of care being followed. Many HISs have a module that identifies the patient's illness or event and, with criteria already entered into the system, produces a "normal" plan of care for a patient with that particular problem. This automated care planning module saves time and does not allow for forgetfulness or accidents.

## Patient Education

Smart consumers are demanding more information on their illnesses, and on the best ways that they can participate in the care process. Consequently, patient education systems are now found not only in the hospital setting but also in physicians' offices. Physicians see the system as contributing to the continual efforts to improve health care and trim costs. Computer-based patient education should be user-friendly and implemented in such a way that physicians, nurses, and office staff can deliver materials in a fast and uncomplicated manner.

Five reasons an automated system is better than a paper system are as follows (Siwicki, 1997):

1. Provides ability to customize the educational documents
2. Eliminates inventory and ordering costs associated with paper-based systems

3. Reduces search times and improves access to all patient education materials
4. Eliminates the need for office space devoted to storage
5. Encourages greater use of patient education by caregivers because it is easy to use

Internet access to patient education materials is also available. This is a sampling of free Internet sites available to health care professionals and consumers:

- **www.achoo.com**

  Features a health care dictionary and is billed as a "health care information jump point"

- **www.mediscene.com**

  A patient education center developed by Al Davies, MD, director of the critical care medicine training program at Baylor College of Medicine

- **www.usaol.com/dol/forpatient.html**

  Doctor on-line, from USA Online, Inc.

- **nhic-nt.health.org/**

  The United States Department of Health and Human Services' National Health Information Center

## Laboratory Systems

An automated laboratory system integrated into the health care organization improves productivity and responsiveness to physician and nurse inquiries. Improvements are noted in the following areas (Ericson, 1995):

- **Multitasking.** The technician can perform several tasks from the same screen.
- **Integration.** This provides physicians with a means of viewing laboratory results with easy access to patient records.
- **Ease of Use.** There are flexible systems using several input devices: keyboard, pen light, or mouse.

The newest idea in laboratory systems is the ability to test blood at the point of care (POC) or the bedside. The systems consist of a handheld device that tests the blood the same way the test is performed in the laboratory. For the laboratory, this sharply reduces the number of handling steps and levels of the organization associated with a typical laboratory test. By streamlining the administration of the test and the reporting process, and integrating with the health care clinical system, the POC systems significantly reduce turnaround time, labor, and the potential for error (Winner, 1995).

## Radiology Systems

Radiology applications challenge the performance of the platform, display, and networking vendors. The applications demand faster systems with increased power and higher resolution monitors, and most of all, the systems must be cost-effective (Braly, 1996). Most vendors offering radiology information systems offer a full line of capabilities. The most common systems include:

- Ad hoc/query report generation
- Film location and tracking
- Radiology order entry and results reporting
- Electronic signature
- Image storage/retrieval
- Inventory control
- Utilization review reports

Some systems also offer digital dictation interfaces. There is a variety of operating platforms from which to choose, such as IBM, UNIX, Windows, Window NT, and DOS.

## Practice Management System

The independent practitioner's office is rapidly disappearing, replaced by networks of physician practices managed by group corporations, management services organizations (MSOs), and integrated delivery systems (IDSs). The success in this movement will be seen in the reduction of overhead administrative costs for the individual practitioner. To make this a reality, automated systems must:

- Enable all practices to share common information about each health plan
- Eliminate redundancy and ensure consistency
- Calculate expected reimbursement for many managed care plans
- Support the unlimited number of fee schedules, which can include provider, health plan, location and service, resource-based relative value studies (RBRVS), sliding scale, per diem, per case, and capitated methods (Solomon, 1997)

Many of the steps involved in a patient encounter that previously took place in the back office now can be accomplished as a part of the front office scheduling and check in/out process.

## Pharmacy

Every detail of drug therapy for the patient is important. The first generation pharmacy systems assisted with medication floor stock replacement and charging. This improved efficiency, accountability, and control of access. The "patient profile" was added in the next generation to limit the selection of items to those ordered for a patient, either through a pharmacy system interface or directly into the system. This addition eliminated the traditional cart fill and reduced medication errors.

The newest pharmacy design is a software application to automate all tasks involved in administration, documentation, alerts, outcome requirements, new order verification, critical dosing, and stat doses. Pharmacy automation has been shown to reduce medication errors, decrease duplication of paperwork, and increase flexibility of scheduling, documentation, and charge capture.

## Telemedicine

Providers with telemedicine capabilities are serving rural and underserved areas. Telemedicine speeds access to specialists and improves health care. It is also cutting costs. Telemedicine software transmits medical images over telephone lines from one computer to another. The software displays the images and enables a specialist at the hospital and a remote physician to communicate in real time by enabling the caregivers to see each other's drawings and notes made directly on the image displayed on the computer screen.

To make these systems work, it is recommended that the provider have at least a Pentium 133 PC with a video card, a two-gigabyte hard drive, and a seventeen-inch high-resolution monitor. To create the photographs, the provider must use a colposcope. This device is something like a microscope on a stick. A colposcope enables the physician to focus on an area of the body, magnify the view, then press one of two buttons to create an image. One button activates a video link and that creates a still image from the video. The other button activates a 35-millimeter camera that takes a picture of the physician's view through the colposcope. Images can be transferred within minutes, and the two providers can be talking on a separate telephone line. Consultations can be done in record time with no travel for either the specialist or the patient.

## Home Care

Many home care agencies have already automated financial operations, including billing, and are seeing positive results. Home care nurses are making use of handheld and laptop computers to gather assessment data. Downloading information over the telephone makes it easy for physicians and nurse practitioners to monitor care given in the home setting.

Most home care agencies are anxious to ensure their systems are compatible with those of the larger health systems. In addition, oxygen companies, durable medical equipment companies, infusion programs, and home care agencies are all striving to develop a standard set of definitions and standard set rates. Automation will help them do this (Cross, 1997).

## Patient Scheduling

One of the advantages of a centralized scheduling system is that appointments can be made at any point in the health care organization. When an appointment is made or changed, the system can automatically send an appointment letter or reminder to the patient. In advance of the appointment, lists of names can be printed and medical records gathered. Comprehensive information about past and future appointments can be analyzed for planning purposes (Lee & Millman, 1995). Key measurements of success are:

- The number and type of rescheduled tests
- The level of scheduling efficiency, for example, first call, schedule with five minutes
- Patient and physician satisfaction
- Scheduling and point-of-service time delay

To enable the right services to be provided at the right level of care with minimal inconvenience and delay for both patients and providers, clinical and management information systems linking all providers at all sites must be developed (Kastens, 1996).

## Acuity Systems

Acuity reflects the amount of nursing time a patient will require, which is dependent on the care the patient needs. Patients are classified by tasks needed. Classification translated into work equals nursing acuity (Saba & McCormick, 1995). Software programs compute staff needs, allocate staff, and produce management reports. They will also report on staff illnesses and absences, overtime, and other programmable elements.

Currently, the software is retrospective in nature. In the decade ahead, acuity, classification, and intensity systems with better control of standardization and comparison between health care organizations will have to be developed (Finnegan, Abel, & Dobler, 1993).

# REFERENCES

Bishop, P. (1986). *Fifth generation computers; concepts, implementations and uses.* New York: Wiley.

Bowden, B. V. (Ed.) (1953). *Faster than thought.* Lanham, MD: Pitman.

Braly, D. (1996). Radiology systems continue pushing technology envelope. *Health Management Technology, 17*(12), 51–53.

Cook, M., & Mayers, M. (1981). Computer-assisted data base for nursing research. In H. Werley & M. Grier (Eds.), *Nursing information systems.* New York: Springer.

Cross, M. (1997). Home care providers turn to automation to improve efficiency. *Health Data Management, 18*(12), 67–71.

Darnell, T. (1996). Materials management systems: All about controlling costs. *Health Management Technology, 17*(13), 15–17.

Ericson, K. (1995). Serving clients in the lab. *Healthcare Informatics, 12*(8), 72–78.

Finnegan, S. A., Abel, M., & Dobler, T., et al. (1993). Automated patient acuity: Linking nursing systems and quality measurement with patient outcomes. *Journal of Nursing Administration, 23*(5), 62–71.

Goedert, J. (1996). Tracking electronic claims growth. *Health Data Management, 4*(11), 73–75.

Hanson, R. L. (1993). Computerized staff scheduling: Opportunities and obstacles to success. *Healthcare Information Management, 7*(3), 3–8.

Hyman, A. (1982). *Charles Babbage: Pioneer of the computer.* Oxford: University Press.

Kastens, J. (1996). Automate simplicity to cut costs. *Health Management Technology, 17*(11), 47–48.

Lee, N., & Millman, A. (1995). Hospital based computer systems. *British Medical Journal, 311*(7011), 1013–1018.

McCormack, J. (1997). EDI enables big cuts in supply procurement costs. *Health Data Management, 5*(5), 107–111.

Saba, V. A., & McCormick, K. A. (1995). *Essentials of computers for nurses.* New York: McGraw-Hill.

Siwicki, B. (1997). Software, Internet create new avenues for patient education. *Health Data Management, 5*(1), 49–56.

Solomon, M. R. (1997). The elements of a successful practice management system. *Health Management Technology, 18*(2), 96–98.

Straub, K. (1997). Mining for strategically significant financial information. *Health Management Technology, 18*(12), 49–52.

Winner, P. (1995). Streamlining lab services: Point of care technology. *Healthcare Informatics, 12*(8), 68–70.

Zielstorff, R. D., McHugh, M. L., & Clinton, J. (1988). *Computer design criteria for systems that support the nursing process.* Kansas City: American Nurses Association.

# CHAPTER

# Defining Roles

Over one hundred years ago, Florence Nightingale wrote *Notes on Nursing: What It Is and What It Is Not*. Even at that time, she alluded to the need for a device that stored data. Nightingale described the work of nurses as "recording the proper selection and administration of diet" (Nightingale, 1946). Seymer (1954) made the observation that "she (Nightingale) stated that the purpose of documenting such observations, was to collect, store, and retrieve data, so that patient care could be managed intelligently."

As the early computer systems were being developed, studies were conducted to determine what aspects of health care would benefit from automation. Because the first computers dealt with mathematical logic, the billing department was the first to make use of the capabilities available. From a clinical vantage point, the data processing department, full of key punch cards and very large noisy machines, was a mysterious place. This function was far removed from the focus of taking care of the sick. The job of data processing was to send out a bill and retrieve payment for the services provided. This job was handled by computer programmers, computer operators, key punch operators, and non–health care managers. Where are we now?

As the computer industry developed health care expertise, the data processing department, focused solely on automating billing, was forced to address and assist other areas of health care. Data processing was renamed information systems, information services, or most recently, information technology. This broader area of expertise needed a leader who could represent the vast potential automation held for the hospital. What was once the role of the data processing manager has now evolved into that of the chief information officer (CIO).

## CHIEF INFORMATION OFFICER (CIO)

Woldring (1996) asks the question, "[D]oes 'CIO' stand for Chief Information Officer or 'Career Is Over?'"

> Confusion is rampant on just what constitutes a CIO. In a survey of over 400 CIO's, only 57% thought of themselves as true CIO's, and only 27% of those, reported directly to top health care administration. A statement concerning the actual power of the CIO is summed up, "we don't state, we suggest" (Woldring, 1996).

Many CIOs reported that they would gladly give up the title, as it makes them an easy target. The longevity of a CIO was shown to be approximately four years. Most enter a health care system as a CIO and leave as a CIO. The myth about this position being a stepping stone to the CEO spot is just that. "They enter the system as an outsider and leave as an outsider" (Carlyle, 1988).

Some of the uncertainty surrounding the true status of the CIO may be the result of ambivalence over the role and the technology the CIO is supposed to champion. Over the last twenty years, the timing of when to "get on board the health care automation train" has been a tricky question. With hospitals in the middle of five-year strategic plans, automation dollars had to wait until the next planning retreat.

There was considerable time spent selling the automation idea. Some chief executive officers (CEOs) needed a new vision to promote, and automation was that breath of fresh air needed to extend their tenure. Automation was growing quickly and steadily in surrounding industries. Even though hospitals were independent for decades, these silos were being toppled in communities all around the country. Hospitals were dependent only on their community reputation concerning quality of patient care and their up-to-date technology. While large teaching and research health care organizations seemed to be moving rapidly toward the forefront of automation technology, even small rural community hospitals were being forced into automation by suppliers, insurance companies, third-party payers, schools, government, and their own staff, whether they were ready for it or not.

Twenty years later, there is still skepticism concerning the need for automation, and if it is needed, to what extent it is needed. Questions that are being asked include: Which service areas would really benefit from automation? Which service areas could change their work flows to allow for automation? What is wrong with the manual systems already in place? What are the benefits and how are they measured? These questions are not easily answered. Administrators see this area as a potential black hole to sink money into, without seeing instant quantitative results.

Ask the question: Does this organization need a CIO? While the job description can be somewhat hazy, the need must be clearly visualized. Is the health care organization information-intensive? Is the health care organization competing with other health care organizations? If the hospital has already implemented some automated systems, are they interfaced, or is there a hodgepodge of stand-alone software applications? Are the systems stagnant while the industry is moving ever forward? Is the health care organization spending large amounts of money on information technology? Is the health care organization spreading out over a wide geographic area? An answer of yes to any of these questions may be a reason to develop a CIO position (Glou, 1995). Identifying and choosing the right person for the job is crucial. Failure to do so can mean a loss of several years to a system's competitive position (Woldring, 1996).

Historically, the job of automation system education fell to the leader of the technicians. This position has had many titles, including data processing manager, manager of information systems, director of information systems, director of information services, director of information technologies, director of information systems/chief information officer, and chief information officer. Each organizational chart varies with the importance placed on this role by the CEO and the hospital board. Along with these titles come different pay scales and different levels of participation in the organization's hierarchy. "Visionaries shape the reality of today into a vision for tomorrow and make the vision come alive. They recognize and use forces that drive change to shape a vision of the future" (Waite, 1989).

If the position reports at a director level, the automation vision is usually at least two levels down from top administration. The CIO position must be a part of the executive team if it is to be optimized (Woldring, 1996). Chief information officers state that "we don't control the information, we make it flow" (Carlyle, 1988). If the health care organization truly holds the information management vision with high regard, the CIO position should act as a right hand to the CEO and the chief operating officer (COO). The person in this position should have a seat on the highest councils and should have an intimate understanding of, and active participation in designing, the organization's strategic plan.

How many hospitals are configured this way? Experts tell us there are not many. Why is that? Currently, few individuals fit the position, and few organizations allow their CIOs to meet their full potential.

Covey (1989) stated:

[I]n a visionary role, a leader must not only be excited about the possibilities, they must be able to communicate and make the uneducated see the vision and be comfortable with it.

Effective management without effective leadership is like straightening the deck chairs on the Titanic.

Leadership is setting the vision that is to be achieved. No management success can compensate for failure in leadership.

Information technology is a science that is difficult for the uninitiated to understand. Information becomes available when an access code is entered into a terminal. But issues concerning how it got there, storage capacity, the speed at which data is processed, how data become information, and a million other questions can be intimidating. What makes these things happen? We cannot see or touch it. Data elements cannot be seen moving around. The computer appears to be a static object. Feedback mechanisms have to be deliberately programmed into the systems we use to let us know there is actually work going on. Technology today can be difficult to comprehend, let alone discuss with the uninitiated. It takes a very good communicator to educate the leaders of our health care organizations to a level of comprehension at which solid visionary decisions concerning information technology can be made. Unfortunately, the person who understands the technology is often a very poor communicator.

Historically, CIOs came from a technical background. They usually possessed a formal computer or engineering education at a bachelor's or master's level. Somewhere along the way, they stumbled into management and into a health care setting. While software applications were unique to the situations, data processing departments across the business community were similar in the activities they performed. Early CIOs never had a clinical background. In a technical sense, although they were working in a hospital, they could have been working and managing a data processing department in any industry.

The most promising applicant, looking at a current health care CIO position, would be a person who has straddled the worlds of business, technology, and health care and has aligned all three (Bunschoten, 1996; Pemberton, 1992). Today, CIOs must make the leap across all boundaries in the health care arena:

> They must possess a very clear understanding of the newest technological advances that could concern and assist in the health care industry. They must understand and be a visionary about hardware, software, and connectivity issues. "Information management is not a basement function any more" (Bunschoten, 1996).

The CIO must be an educator and a clear communicator of difficult concepts to all levels of staff and community. Pemberton (1992) suggests:

> [D]on't assume the senior executives are automatically interested in information technology, get their attention first. Get to the bottom line quickly; never take more than twenty minutes to explain anything; avoid technical terminology; and finally, concentrate on the big picture.

According to Siwicki (1995), CIOs must possess exemplary business skills in regard to the management of both people and information—they must understand fiscal appropriation and be able to communicate and lead people. Bunschoten (1996) states that CIOs must "exhibit leadership qualities and learn how to ask the right questions."

The clinical component of health care information technology must be explored and understood at a high level by CIOs. The business of hospitals, hospital systems, and health care enterprises is maintaining health. Those in the highest positions in the corporation must have a good understanding of the important tools to support this business (Bunschoten, 1996).

The CIO is a key player in any future information technologies the health care organization will use. The CIO's insight into the potential and the limitations of each future application can make a crucial difference in the organization's positioning. The CIO's role is to "interpret business requirements, do the high-level planning, and make sure the funding, direction and vision all mesh with each other" (Bazzoli, 1996; Bunschoten, 1996). By interweaving the four areas of technology, communication, business and health care, the CIO has the knowledge and experience to take the lead in these situations and be successful in fulfilling the corporate strategic goals.

In 1995, Woldring studied the CIO role and discovered a recurring pattern of turnover. With good information about what makes a CIO successful, why does the health care industry see such a large turnover in CIO positions? In Woldring's study, the three patterns discussed in the following text emerged consistently.

**Pattern 1: The Technical CIO.** Organizations that are relatively new to automation or just decide to elevate the data processing manager position to a CIO role are drifting into unknown territory. Often the top administrators in health care corporations see the need for information technology but do not have the expertise to tackle the issues themselves. They decide they need a CIO. Several candidates are brought in to interview. The most capable candidates ask about the reporting structure. They are looking for a reporting structure that allows this position to sit with the top administrative team. The top executives, not envisioning the role of CIO as being part of their senior executive team, see this type of candidate as too aggressive and demanding. The administrative board chooses someone who expects the CIO role to be a supportive one, with a reporting relationship lower in the organization (Woldring, 1996).

A couple years will pass, and the senior executive team will find themselves with a CIO who is largely technology-driven, instead of business-driven. The person in this position has not had the chance for input into or understanding of corporate strategic goals and objectives. So the information technology (IT) department's budget increases, and implementations are never adequate or fast enough. The technical CIO is always playing catch-up. There is dissatisfaction concerning slow projects among line management, who repeat their frustrations to their bosses. The CIO may argue that the corporate culture needs to change and that the information technology department is different from the rest of the organization. If the senior administration is unwilling to hear this, the relationship deteriorates, and the result is inevitable.

**Pattern 2: The Business CIO.** Because of the failing efforts of the technical CIO, the next CIO in this organization may be an internal executive who does not have technology experience, but who does have well-established relationships with peers and a good understanding of the health care business. In some cases, this person is used to bring the information technology department costs under control and to refocus the efforts of information technology on projects that will bring quick results within acceptable time frames.

As the business CIO introduces ways to contain costs, she is alienated from the information technology professionals. The information technology staff respects the CIO's personal qualities and business knowledge, but they are skeptical about her technical leadership abilities. Believing that cost containment means limited career opportunities, the most promising of the information technology staff look for other jobs. Some leave and create holes in service. Replacements often need to be trained and have less expertise, costing more time and creating more information technology inefficiency. New recruits are cautious when they find out the business is in the midst of massive change and may drop out of the interviewing process.

Woldring (1996) states that one of two things will happen to the business CIO. In scenario 1, in the short-term, information technology costs will come under control, and operating results from existing applications and investments will improve. The focus on present costs, however, reduces the organization's ability to build for the future. Senior administration realizes that although the business CIO has done her job, future vision is lacking, and they need someone who can rebuild the information technology organization. The business CIO is rewarded with another business job, usually within the organization, and the search for the new information technology CIO begins.

In scenario 2, the situation can get even more complicated. The business CIO can see there is need for future information technology development, but because she does not have expertise in the technological aspects, she delegates responsibility to existing professionals. This removes her from actual projects, and she is dependent on others who may not have the right business background and corporate strategic vision to ask the right questions. As problems accumulate, this CIO begins to feel the pressure of this lack of knowledge. Often she makes an effort to cope, but in the end, the individual moves on, and the search for the CIO starts again.

**Pattern 3: The Successful CIO Leaves.** This organization has a successful CIO, and the senior administration understands the importance of the CIO role. They have embraced the CIO as a member of their team, and all have a clear understanding of both the accountabilities and the competencies of the role. This CIO performs as expected. This person's competencies match the requirements well, and the information technology projects are focused. An infrastructure evolves, and costs are directly related to the overall impact on the system. The line managers are happy and are rewarded for improved operating results. Information technology is clearly in a support role. Most of the rewards, incentives, raises, and bonuses, however, go to the operations side of the organization. This CIO may begin to feel that information technology is a dead-end job. She will take another position as opportunities are offered.

So, what is the answer? The needs are clear. The senior administration must have very clear expectations concerning information technology and its contribution to the strategic future of the organization. Once the competencies are defined and agreed upon, there must be a match with the successful CIO. The leader of information technology will need access to, and participation in, discussions concerning corporate strategic planning. This means the CIO must be a part of the senior administrative team. "This is an information-intensive business, and the ability to have the right information available, in the right place, at the right time, warrants having a CIO at the table, in the highest parts of the organization" (Bunschoten, 1996).

In 1995, Hewlett-Packard did a leadership study, asking about the most important skills a CIO could possess (Bunschoten, 1996). Six skills were reported upon and ranked as follows:

- Business strategy development      49%
- Consensus building      19%
- Creative problem solving      14%
- Ability to motivate      7%
- Interpersonal skills      7%
- Negotiating skills      4%

Ruffin (1996) suggests that "in the next century, clinicians, most of whom will be physician executives, will lead the operation of and investment in, information and communication systems for most health care organizations." This is due to the "substantial financial incentives to invest in clinically oriented information technologies, to measure and manage clinical details about patients in electronic form, to alert clinicians to practice guidelines, and to increase the efficiency of data communication about patients to clinicians in their homes and offices" (Ruffin, 1996). This is an interesting opinion. The physician executive, however, would appear to bring at least the same liabilities to the position as the business CIO.

Traditionally, clinical information systems have not played a leading role in decision support for health care organizations. Finance and accounting applications have been used exclusively by administration for decision making. This custom must change to support clinical quality improvement, to develop practice guidelines, and to standardize the profiling of clinicians' practice habits. No other department in the health care arena is in a better position than information systems to play this crucial role. This department should seek out opportunities to help clinicians and managers improve their work.

Usually, the information systems department maintains financial data processing and decision support systems. Sometimes it maintains the clinical transaction processing, such as laboratory, pharmacy, and radiology systems. What it usually does not maintain is departmental data repositories, such as tumor, transplant, and trauma registries, and databases used to record clinical treatments and outcomes of patients. The keepers of these clinical databases usually are not included in the planning or implementation of information systems but are left on their own to find their way (Ruffin, 1996).

All these independent decisions made by various departments lead to the situation found at most hospitals today—many separate and narrowly focused software applications. This makes consistent data definitions within an organization almost impossible. No standard covers all situations. ICD-9-CM codes and SNOMED III are helpful but are not all-inclusive. Human intervention is necessary. Standards need to be adopted through multidisciplinary consensus.

The clinical CIO or an informatics nursing specialist (INS) may be an answer. The information systems CIO must supervise and manage the organization that installs, implements, maintains, and upgrades electronic information and communication technologies. A clinical CIO or INS could lead clinicians to successful data standardization, collection, and analysis for clinical quality improvement and outcomes management (Ruffin, 1996). This position would be devoted to developing expertise in data collection and profiling physicians and nursing care, using quality improvement exercises (Simpson, 1994).

As the management of information becomes more intricate and insidious, perhaps there is a place for both the successful CIO and the clinically based practitioner. While the stand-alone clinical CIO is an interesting idea, for all the reasons that were discussed in Patterns 1–3, the clinical CIO would fail also. The CIO who will succeed in the twenty-first century has to be multifaceted and will need to surround herself with knowledgeable support staff. Hospital organizational structures will need to make room at the table for one more and share their corporate vision and goals. This position will only get bigger as health care automation expands. It will take a very sharp person to make it successful.

Ideally, the CIO should manage all information and the tools that assist in managing the information. The CIO should:

- Define the information to be used in the organization
- Set information policy and standards
- Maintain management control over all information resources—not just the data and information stored on computers, but the nonautomated information that is stored in file cabinets, libraries, and manuals

Technology is the focus of the CIO's job. Today it is common for the CIO to have control over the technology, but very few CIOs have total control over all information resources. It is important that the CIO have knowledge of the technology and also have the ability to speak in terms of information capabilities to the layperson (Davenport, 1995).

## FILLING THE CIO ROLE

How can we get the right person in the right position? It is difficult to always select the right candidate for each position, but it is possible to determine some general characteristics that are needed. Mapping out the CIO role is helpful. When hiring for any position, it is useful to review the four elements that go into any position:

**Accountabilities.** Define what is expected of the individual. These expectations come from an organization's general objectives and working structure. They should be consistent across many positions.

**Competencies.** Indicate what an individual is able to do. Competencies detail a person's abilities and experiences as seen by others, describe past behaviors and achievements, and predict future performance on the basis of these past behaviors.

**Performance Measures.** Rate how well predetermined expectations are being met. Both the manager and employee, as a way of measuring and determining success, agree upon each performance measure. Essentially, performance measures create effective job descriptions. They move performance expectations from generalizations to the specific results desired from each individual.

**Authority.** Define what decisions an individual can make, and what resources—dollars, people, and other assets—the individual can use in achieving her performance goals and targets.

The interrelationship of these four elements allows an organization to effectively evaluate a person's job performance by creating an accountability outline (Woldring, 1996).

The CIO must be willing to:

- Put the health care organization's needs ahead of her own information technology department needs or technology direction
- Demonstrate consistent integrity and loyalty to the enterprise in general, rather than to information technology
- Build and maintain effective working relationships within the organization
- Set up and monitor an internal performance map that measures the progress of information technology in business terms

- Understand the health care organization's operations and its strategic direction so the information technology development efforts are focused on projects that deliver real value to the organization
- Keep the organization's senior administrative team informed about the potential operational and financial impact of new information technology developments
- Build and maintain an information and technology infrastructure that contributes to the business in the long term

## CIO'S ACCOUNTABILITIES AND COMPETENCIES

Building a matrix is an effective method of developing a profile on the individual who is likely to succeed. Studies have found that eleven core competencies in general business management, and eight core competencies in clinical areas, are required for a CIO to be successful (Simpson, 1994; Woldring, 1996).

From a general business management perspective, CIOs should be able to:

1. Set challenging, concrete goals and objectives for themselves and for others
2. Find better, more cost-effective methods of completing tasks
3. Seize the opportunity to act before being asked to act or forced to act by events
4. Seek information from many different sources
5. Determine ways to have an impact on or persuade an individual or group
6. Build a rapport with people through informal contacts carried out in day-to-day work
7. Build long-term alliances with others, both inside and outside the organization, to help achieve goals and objectives
8. Communicate with clients, both internal and external to the organization, clarifying their needs and taking steps to involve them in activities that meet the clients' short- and long-term goals
9. Solicit input from others who are affected by planned information technology activities
10. Understand a complex task and process the concept by breaking it down into manageable parts in a systematic and detailed way
11. Apply professional or technical knowledge in day-to-day work

The eight clinical core competencies to be expected in successful CIOs are:

1. Understanding that information technology is an interdepartmental process and what that means
2. Understanding the important role clinical data must and should play in the development of an information management system

3. Understanding how computers and telecommunications technology can be used for staff development and clinical practice enhancement
4. Understanding how clinical decision support systems can be used for strategic planning
5. Understanding the ethical issues regarding information technology, security, and confidentiality
6. Knowing how to evaluate, select, and manage the services of information management consultants
7. Understanding how to use information technology for data collection for regulatory compliance
8. Understanding market forces, vendor marketing techniques, and emerging technologies for future decision making

## Performance Measures

Performance measures are determined after the position has been filled. The new CIO and her administrator should spend the time and effort needed to decide on the expectations and targets for the position for a specified period. Specific performance measures may take on the goals and objectives format, with dates and amounts of completion noted. These performance measures are an effective way for administration to make sure the CIO is staying on track with the corporate strategic plan, and they give the CIO a specific path to follow.

## Authority

During the creation of performance measures, take into consideration the accountabilities and competencies the new CIO already possesses. Talk about the accountabilities and competencies the CIO must work on, and how specifically she might accomplish these goals. This is the time to remind both the new CIO and the senior administrator of the CIO's span of authority over resources—such as dollars, people, and other assets—that she may use to achieve her performance targets.

We recommend that a new CIO and her immediate administrator discuss one of these performance measures each month. The continuous review and dialogue about these goals and objectives will strengthen the likelihood that they will be met and that both the administration and the CIO will be successful.

Today's CIOs must have clinical knowledge or an informatics nursing specialist (INS), a clinical liaison, to assist them in their decisions. Ruffin (1996) reports on a survey that addressed the issues commonly faced by a CIO in a integrated health care organization. These issues were rated in regard to the importance of clinical assistance with each topic, using the indicators low, moderate, and high. The results are presented in Figure 2–1. With

| | |
|---|---|
| • Selection of clinical transaction systems for basic clinical information collection and communication: laboratory, radiology, order entry and results reporting, enterprise wide scheduling, pharmacy | Moderate |
| • Selection of managed care information systems for PHOs, MSOs, and IPAs to allow them to manage inpatient and outpatient care, develop capitation contracts, and to collect data for retrospective study for physicians' practice habits | Moderate |
| • Selection of standardized office practice information systems to lead physicians to standard patient accounting and computer-based medical record systems | High |
| • Design and implementation of a wide-area communications network linking work stations in all facilities of the organization with standardized clinical and financial transaction systems | Low |
| • Design and implementation of a regional communications network linking physicians' homes and offices to electronic data about patients, electronic scheduling of services, and electronic mail to payers and other physicians | High |
| • Upgrading of financial information systems (primarily patient accounting) for management of managed care contracts | Low |
| • Procurement and implementation of computer-based patient records for intensive care units and emergency departments, the functional requirements of which may not be satisfied by patient care systems for hospitals | High |
| • Procurement and implementation of cost accounting systems for hospitals and group practices to enable managers to identify their "true" costs of operations | High |
| • Design and implementation of a telemedicine network for communication by clinicians in real time and multimedia electronic mail to expedite clinical consultations | High |
| • Design and implementation of a home page, with derivative documents, on the Internet to be used by the community for access to general health information, details about clinicians, triage algorithms for patients, and schedules of clinical services | Moderate |
| • Leadership for information systems planning and budgeting for the next five years | High |
| • Design, funding, and implementation of a relational corporate data warehouse to support retrospective data analysis for health services and clinical research | High |
| • Creation of a team of health services research specialists to analyze data from the data warehouse and support clinical data analysis and risk adjustment by various managerial and clinical groups within the organization | High |
| • Tailoring of computer-based patient record systems to meet the needs of clinicians, physicians, nurses, and others in ambulatory and inpatient settings | High |

**Figure 2–1** Issues facing CIOs: Importance of clinical assistance

| | |
|---|---|
| • Participation in managed care contracting initiatives to make certain that terms of contracts that affect information systems can be accomplished by the health care organization | High |
| • Development of training programs for all clinicians, physicians, nurses, physical therapists, pharmacists, and others—to learn to use computer-based patient records selected for office practices and inpatient settings | High |
| • Participation of the organization in national data collection initiatives, standardizing and producing data for national benchmarking programs (C/FIS of Voluntary Hospitals of America, IMSystems of JCAHO, HEDIS of NCQA, MQISS of HCFA, and PROs) devoted to accreditation, quality improvement, and outcomes management | High |
| • Definition of functional requirements and procurement of information systems, such as registries for cardiovascular surgery and transplant surgery, for clinical departments of group practices and hospitals | High |
| • Standardization of software for electronic mail, groupware, and access to the Internet so that the organization can offer to its employees and on-line customers a standardized interface to all electronic information | Low |
| • Leadership of health services research staff for data analysis to support clinical quality improvement and outcomes management and practice guidelines development | High |

**Figure 2–1** (continued)

these survey results in mind, and knowing that there are very few CIOs with clinical background, let us look at a new specialty role for nurses.

## INFORMATICS NURSING SPECIALIST (INS)

With the advent of automation creeping into every aspect of the health care arena, nurses have been sought as the experts on what a clinical information system should contain. The nurse is usually closer to patient care issues than any other health care professional. Graves and Osbolt (1992) point out, "Nursing informatics has been defined as a combination of computer science, information science and nursing science designed to assist in the management and processing of nursing data, information and knowledge to support the practice of nursing and the delivery of nursing care."

The American Nurses Association (ANA), the national professional organization for nurses, serves as the certification agency for informatics nursing. The ANA (1994) has defined informatics as "the activities involved in identifying, naming, organizing, grouping, collecting, processing, analyzing, storing, retrieving or managing data and information." Nursing informatics is a specialty that "integrates nursing science, computer science, and information science in identifying, collecting, processing, and managing data and information to support nursing practice, administration, education, research, and the expansion of nursing knowledge" (ANA, 1994).

## INS Core Competencies

There are many forward-thinking nurse managers who understand how important it is for the profession of nursing to incorporate technology into nursing practice. It is no longer true that the person "who controls the purse strings, controls all"; now the person "who controls information, controls just as much" (Simpson, 1994). Few nurse administrators in service today have core competencies in nursing informatics. This is to be expected. There are very few graduate programs or certification opportunities currently. Judith Ronald, EdD, RN, FAAN, a leading nursing informatics researcher, has put together the following list of core competencies for nursing informatics:

- Understand the basic "tools" and terminology of the trade and have some experience with computers and information technology
- Understand how information technology can help with decision making and strategic planning at the executive level
- Understand how to actively and effectively participate in the evaluation, selection, implementation, and maintenance of a health care organization's information system
- Understand that information technology is an interdepartmental process and what that means to the nursing department as a whole
- Understand the important role nursing data must play in the development or selection of a hospital information system
- Understand how computers and telecommunications technology can be used for staff development and clinical practice enhancement
- Understand how decision support systems can be used for strategic planning
- Understand the ethical issues regarding information technology, security, and confidentiality
- Know how to evaluate, select, and manage the services of information technology consultants
- Understand how to use information technology for data collection for regulatory compliance
- Understand market forces, vendor marketing techniques, and emerging technologies for future decision making

So, how can nurses become familiar with these core competencies? They can learn from the information technology executives. Sit on the information management steering committee at your institution. Get involved in meeting the JCAHO information management standards. Read articles about information technology, attend educational seminars, ask vendors questions, and get involved in ANA and professional computer organizations, for example, the Hospital Information Management System Society (HIMSS) or the Council on Hospital Information Management (CHIM). For nurses, this is the time to brush up on, and continue to strengthen, their knowledge of nursing informatics.

## Certification Process

To sit for the national certification examination, INSs must meet the following qualifications:

- Currently hold an active registered nursing license in the United States or its territories; and
- Hold a baccalaureate or higher degree in nursing; and
- Have practiced as a licensed registered nurse for a minimum of 2 years and meet the following in their current practice:
  — Have practiced at least 2,000 hours in the field of informatics nursing within the past 5 years; or
  — Have completed at least 12 semester hours of academic credits in informatics in a graduate program in nursing and have practiced a minimum of 1,000 hours in informatics nursing within the past 5 years; and
- Have had 20 contact hours of continuing education applicable to the specialty area within the past 2 years. Documentation of continuing education must be submitted. Author/presenter credits are allowable but can account for not more than one-half of the contact hour requirement. Author's work must be in a refereed publication. Combinations of continuing education and academic credit hours are acceptable. Contact hour credit will be allowed for attendance at professional meetings that include content appropriate to informatics nursing practice. Independent study, which has been approved for continuing education or academic credit, is also allowed (American Nurses Credentialing Center, 1995).

The certification examination covers the following areas of expertise:

- System analysis and design
- System implementation and support
- System testing and evaluation
- Human factors
- Computer technology
- Information/database management

• Professional practice/trends and issues
• Theories

The ANA and the experts in the field have discovered that some valuable skills to possess before taking the examination include: competency in hardware and software development cycles; functional hardware skills, such as installation and maintenance of basic software packages; knowledge of system integration issues; knowledge of computer programming languages; Internet vocabulary; and some experience with project management strategies commonly used for implementation of large software applications.

## Functional Responsibilities of an INS in a Health Care Organization

Nationwide, there are a variety of reporting structures in which INSs can find themselves involved. At some health care organizations, the INS will have an office in the information technology area and report to the CIO. In another scenario, the INS may report directly to the chief nursing officer and be housed within the nursing department. In either case, the INS should be a member of the information management steering committee, where the INS, as nurse liaison, can offer assistance with decisions surrounding automation in specific health care environments.

The nurse liaison has the background to determine the work of "nursing." Should there be a question concerning how an application will affect nursing's work flow, the INS will investigate the impact and report the findings to the work group or responsible team. She will be the point person for questions and negotiations with nursing as a department. During work group meetings, an INS has the ability to construct work relationships by the use of flow diagramming to demonstrate the impacts of applications. This position provides the expertise to determine the automation capabilities needed in a health care organization.

In balancing her attendance at the information management steering committee meetings, the INS should also be a member of the nursing executive council. It is imperative that she be active in both the clinical and information management departments. Because the INS has both global and specific information concerning both specialties, the person in this position can answer many questions concerning both current and future automation and clinical plans.

### INS Assisting with System Selection Process

The Joint Commission on Accreditation of Healthcare Organizations (JCAHO) standards support the use of interdisciplinary teams in the selection process of health care information technology. During the selection process, the INS investigates all possible solutions, including manual solutions, to determine the new capabilities that are needed in each health care area. This role, which is similar to the investigation process that must be completed before the purchase of any new software product, includes:

- Review of the corporate strategic plan to find evidence of need for a new application and for specific guidelines and strategies concerning new software application purchases
- Review of current literature, attendance at trade shows, and interviews of associates to determine "best of breed" in software that may meet the organization's needs
- Knowledge of how to develop a request for information (RFI) that will be used to gather information concerning specific software vendors
- Ability to set a realistic application search schedule that includes vendors that can meet the organization's needs
- Calling of potential vendors to verify their interest in the organization's project
- Distribution of an RFI with specific instructions and date for return
- Review of the RFI answers and the ability to rank the top five vendors
- Development of a request for proposal (RFP) to further clarify the specific capabilities needed in the health care environment
- Distribution of the RFP with specific instructions and date for return
- Review of the RFP answers and ability to rank the top three vendors
- Scheduling live on-site demonstrations for each of the final three vendors
- Invitation of appropriate people to review each vendor and evaluate the software capabilities directly after the demonstration
- Review and tabulation of the evaluation scores after each demonstration
- Presentation of the findings to the information management steering committee
- Escorting a representative health care organization group to a similar organization situation for a live-site visit
- Scheduling and attendance at the contract negotiations of the selected vendor

## *Nurse Educator*

The INS serves as the liaison between the technical and the clinical professionals. The person in this position reviews, schedules, monitors, and supervises any computer training needed. The INS supports the clinical staff in their efforts to attend training, and evaluates the results of the training afterward. If there are special circumstances, for example, special needs for any employee, the INS proposes solutions. The INS acts as the staff's advocate if problems arise in any training situation.

Along with formal computer training, the INS is responsible for informal training and on-the-spot problem solving. If a clinical manager is having difficulty with a spreadsheet application and needs assistance, the INS may be a resource. In a variety of settings, the INS can shed light on any automation issues as they arise. The INS will have insight into the corporate strategic plan and the vision of the health care organization's future. If used correctly, the INS will eliminate many difficult situations by using her knowledge of the clinical aspects of health care and the automation opportunities to make the clinical aspects more manageable.

The roles of professionals working in the health care organization's information technology department are varied and multidimensional. There is a place for the clinician wanting to move into the nursing informatics field, and there is a need for leadership and expertise from the CIO. Rarely can this be the same person, but two professionals can work in collaboration. Regardless of the structure, these jobs must be done effectively and efficiently with the overall good of the organization in mind.

# REFERENCES

American Nurses Association. (1994). *The scope of practice for nursing informatics.* Washington, DC: Author.

American Nurses Credentialing Center. (1995). *Informatics certification catalog.* Washington, DC: Author.

Bazzoli, F. (1996). Getting the job done. *Health Data Management 4*(7), 25.

Bunschoten, B. (1996). From the back room to the board room. *Health Data Management, 1996*(2), 33–41.

Carlyle, R. E. (1988). CIO misfit or misnomer? *Datamation, 34*(15), 50.

Covey, S. R. (1989). *The seven habits of highly effective people.* New York: Simon & Schuster.

Davenport, T. H. (1995). A day in the future of an information executive. *Computerworld, 1*(4), 3–7.

Glou, A. B. (1995). Do you need a CIO? It depends. Here's how to decide. *Inc., 95*(3), 23.

Graves, J. R., & Osbolt, J. G. (1995). Clinical nursing informatics—developing tools for knowledge workers. *Nursing Clinics of North America, 28*(2), 407–417.

Joint Commission on Accreditation of Healthcare Organizations. (1998). *Comprehensive accreditation manual for hospitals.* Oakbrook Terrance, IL: Author.

Nightingale, F. (1946). *Notes on nursing, What it is and what it is not* (facsimile of the 1859 edition). Philadelphia: Lippincott.

Parker, C. D., & Gassert, C. (1996). JCAHO's management of information standards; the role of the informatics nurse specialist. *Journal of Nursing Administration, 26*(6), 13–15.

Pemberton, J. M. (1992). Will the real CIO please stand up? *Records Management Quarterly, 26*(4), 40.

Ruffin, M. (1996, February). Health care bytes: Many chief information officers will be physician executives. *Physician Executive, 22*(2).

Seymer, L. R. (1954). *Selected writings of Florence Nightingale.* New York: Macmillan.

Simpson, R. L. (1993). Shifting perceptions: Defining nursing informatics, as a clinical specialty. *Nursing Management, 24*(12), 20–21.

Simpson, R. L. (1994). Nursing informatics core competencies. *Nursing Management, 25*(5), 18–20.

Siwicki, B. (1995). Where does the CIO fit? *Health Data Management, 1995*(9), 71–73.

Waite, R. M. (1989). *The driving forces for change: Nursing vital signs—shaping the profession for the 1990's.* Battle Creek, MI: W. K. Kellogg Foundation.

Woldring, R. (1996). Information technology: Choosing the right CIO. *Business Quarterly, 60*(3).

# CHAPTER

# Defining Direction

Before software applications can be evaluated and implemented, your organization's needs must be identified. Needs are large and small, but in the end they probably have a relationship to the short- and long-term goals and objectives of the organization. If your organization has no plans of becoming part of the managed care business, then there is probably no need for a managed care system. It is always best to take a top down approach to needs assessment (see Figure 3–1).

## CORPORATE STRATEGIC PLAN

The needs assessment process begins with a review of the health care organization's corporate strategic plan. From this plan, which usually covers a three- to five-year period, one can determine the planned direction of the organization. During this review, attempt to identify what the information management function can do to support these corporate goals. Are new services planned? Will additional clinics be built or physician

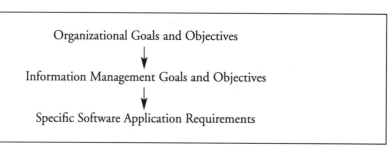

**Figure 3–1** Top down approach to needs assessment (Marreel & McLellan, 1998)

practices added? Will there be a demand for improved and faster decision support information?

Drawing upon the needs identified in the corporate strategic plan, an information management plan that covers the same period as the corporate plan can be developed.

## INFORMATION MANAGEMENT

*Information management* is an important term that has been popularized recently by the Joint Commission on Accreditation of Healthcare Organizations (JCAHO). According to the JCAHO (1998), "Information Management is a *function* focused on meeting the organization's information needs." It is a set of activities and processes. "[T]he goal of Information Management is to obtain, manage, and use information to enhance and improve individual and organizational performance in patient care, governance, management and support processes" (JCAHO, 1998).

Information management is different from information systems in that information systems is an organizational department, while information management is an organizational function. Information management is integral to daily operation. Virtually all the information an organization uses for patient care, governance, management, and support processes, both automated and nonautomated, is included under the information management umbrella. Everyone participates.

## What Kinds of Information?

Examples of the types of information we are concerned with include:

- Patient episodic
- Patient population
- Patient financial
- Quality

- Outcomes
- Decision support
- Media
- Information access and development tools

Data gathering, information gathering, information sharing, information security, and information reporting are all activities and processes that are included within information management. Because of this, virtually everyone in the organization is involved in one way or another with this function. Principal daily participants include: administration, health information management (medical records), information systems, library services, medical staff, and nursing.

## The Information Management Plan

Information is managed in many forms. We receive and communicate information directly by telephone, voice mail, E-mail, and fax. We gather and distribute information on new and returning patients using multipart forms and computer screens. We collect and report on clinical and financial information by both automated and nonautomated means. Every observation that is recorded, every order that is processed, contributes to the collective volume of data and information that is generated on a daily basis in every health care organization. It is the effective and efficient management of that information that is the subject of the information management plan.

From a planning standpoint, therefore, the information management plan tends to be much broader in scope than the information systems plan. In fact, the information systems plan is really a subset of the information management plan. It is imperative that the information systems function be well represented during development of the information management plan.

The purpose of an information management plan is to move the organization forward to an improved state. The information management plan includes both systems and performance improvement goals and objectives. It is both a strategic plan and an action plan.

### *Strategic Component*

The strategic plan defines what it is the organization wants to do, where it wants to go, and what it wants to become. A strategic plan is an outline of an approach, an agenda to be followed. It is all encompassing. There is only one strategic plan. In order to keep a strategic plan viable, there must be a review process in place to keep it up-to-date. So, a strategic plan is never static, it is an ever-evolving document that changes as the needs of the organization change (Palmer & Varnet, 1990).

## Action Component

The action component of the information management plan includes project plans that are developed to accomplish specific objectives in the strategic plan. There will be many action plans within your information management plan. There will be project plans for both systems activities and performance improvement activities. The action plan defines specific tasks, lists target dates, and assigns responsibilities. It deals with specific details that need to be accomplished to reach the goals outlined in the strategic plan.

Using an analogy from frontier days, suppose you have responsibility for shepherding a wagon train going from St. Joseph, Missouri, to Oregon. The purpose, or mission, of your journey is to get the wagon train to Oregon. From a strategic standpoint, there are strategies used to accomplish this mission. If you are the wagon train master, you have an idea, or picture, of your mission, your goals, and the objectives you need to meet to reach those goals and eventually accomplish your mission. In order to begin the trip, specific actions will be required. You can be in Missouri and have a strategic plan, but if you do not have an action plan, you will never get to Oregon—you will never begin your trip. Action plans, particularly those in an information management plan, often take the form of project plans.

## JCAHO Perspective

The JCAHO has provided guidelines on what an information management plan should look like. Keep in mind that your organization does not want to develop an information management plan just as an exercise to satisfy the JCAHO requirements. This should be a planning effort that benefits the operations of your organization. As long as you are at it, however, why not do something that will benefit your hospital accreditation process too? According to JCAHO guidelines, the plan should:

- Define the mission, goals, and objectives for information management
- Clearly identify the health care information management customers
- Assess users' information needs
- Explore ways to improve existing products
- Offer new products and services to meet user needs
- Present evidence that the products are necessary at the level proposed by the plan
- Explain how those products will be packaged and delivered
- Address the four types of information that should be produced: aggregate, patient-specific, comparative, and knowledge-based
- Describe how customer satisfaction will be monitored
- Propose a system to help users maximize the effectiveness of products
- Assess human, technological, and educational resource needs
- Outline a strategy for implementing the plan

## Developing an Information Management Plan

As illustrated in Figure 3–2, there is a hierarchy to an information management plan. The plan is developed from the top down, beginning with the mission statement, followed by the strategies, the goals, the objectives, and detailed action items under each objective. All the elements in the plan, from the mission statement to the detailed action plans, must have three similar characteristics—that is, they should all be specific, measurable, and changeable.

### *Mission Statement*

A mission statement is a statement of your purpose. You go on a mission. You can tell if you are on course or not, because there are implicit and explicit results attached to it. When you describe your mission, you are describing your future and your work.

The mission statement is not written by one person. This is a group effort. Typically, the information management steering committee formalizes the mission statement. This

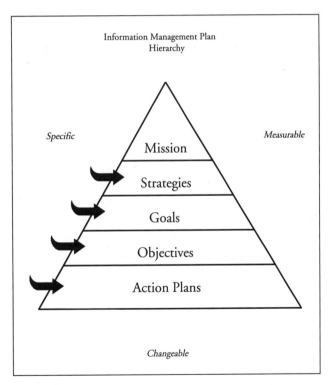

Information Management Plan
Hierarchy

*Specific*                                                    *Measurable*

Mission

Strategies

Goals

Objectives

Action Plans

*Changeable*

**Figure 3–2** Hierarchy of an information management plan (Marreel & McLellan, 1998)

is important because everyone on the committee needs to take ownership of the information management plan. Many people are more comfortable with the concept of an information systems plan than an information management plan. If there is to be consensus within the committee about the future for information management, there first must be consensus on what information management is, and the role that it will play in the future of the organization.

During this process, it is common for each member to have the assignment of writing his own version of a mission statement. By bringing these attempts together, the committee has a place to begin developing a final comprehensive version with which everyone will be satisfied.

A good mission statement answers the following questions:

• What business are we in?
• Where are we going?
• Who are we?
• How do we see ourselves?

The mission statement should be totally understandable by all possible audiences and still be current in three to five years, assuming the philosophy of the organization has not changed. A mission statement need not be long. One or two well-written sentences can be very effective.

When writing a mission statement for the information management plan, first review your corporate strategic mission statement (Marreel & McLellan, 1998). Read it carefully and find the main topics. The following is an example of a corporate mission statement:

> The Hospital Corporation will maintain a leadership position in efficiently providing high-quality medical and health care services to the community. Services will meet identified community needs and shall be provided with concern for our patients and their families. These services will be provided at the lowest possible cost.

> The Corporation will sustain and develop educational programming in medicine, nursing, and health-related professions to promote the highest possible standards of medical care and to maintain the availability of appropriate numbers of quality health employees in the community.

> The Corporation will generate sufficient financial resources to meet the operational needs of services provided and to strategically posture for capital needs, technological advancements, and delivery system enhancements. The Corporation will serve as a responsible employer and participate in the economic and cultural development of the Community.

When you read your own corporate mission statement, make note of the main topics. Remember that the JCAHO (1998) tells us that the goal of information management is to "obtain, manage, and use information to enhance and improve individual and organization performance in patient care, governance, management and support processes."

Using these two sources, the corporate mission statement and the JCAHO statement, you should be able to develop your own information management mission statement. Then, check the result to see whether it clearly answers each of these questions:

- What business are we in?
- Where are we going?
- Who are we?
- How do we see ourselves?
- Will this statement be current in three to five years, assuming the philosophy of the organization has not changed?
- Is this statement totally understandable by all possible audiences?

## Goals

Goals are the issue-specific aims of the organization that allow for the eventual achievement of the mission. Goal setting is a policy-making and agenda-building process that is designed to move the organization to an improved state of readiness or operation.

The wagon train from St. Joseph, Missouri, would certainly develop goals for itself before setting out. One goal might be to begin as soon as they received word from an advance party that the snow melt and spring rains had dried sufficiently to allow passage over muddy trails and across rivers and streams. Other goals might be to reach the area of present-day North Platte, Nebraska, by May 15 and Chimney Rock by June 15. Goals should be major, specific, and measurable.

Three pieces of information are key before you begin developing goals:

1. Knowledge of the long-term direction of the organization
2. Understanding of the framework within which the organization management activities will occur
3. Full appreciation of the organization's continuum of care

The best place to begin is with your corporate strategic plan. Information management goals should be based on corporate goals. Your organization should have a current plan; if not, interview executive-level management. However it is done, determine the long-term goals and objectives of your organization.

Generally, corporate objectives containing an information management component become information management goals. For example, under a corporate goal to "improve the accessibly of our services to the community," one of the objectives may be to open a new clinic in a remote part of town in six months. Based on that *objective,* the information management *goal* should be to "provide the information management capabilities required for operation of the new clinic." Other information management goals should be developed in a similar manner.

## Objectives

Objectives represent the agenda that will be followed to accomplish a goal. There is usually more than one objective under each goal. The only exception to this is when the first objective is to conduct a study to determine the feasibility of, and options for, pursuing a goal. If a viable option is identified, additional objectives are then developed. In the earlier example, the information management goal to "provide the information management capabilities required for operation of the new clinic" would have several objectives. These objectives would be related to the implementation of required hardware and software capabilities, development of new forms, development of procedures, and training of staff. Objectives generally turn into individual projects, each with a project plan and a project team.

When writing objectives, keep them short and to the point. Begin each objective with an action verb. This tends to focus the thought process, avoiding fuzzy objectives. In order to monitor progress, objectives must be clear and measurable. When writing objectives:

- State exactly what must be achieved.
- Make them specific and measurable, and clearly identify the "what" and "when."
- Start each objective with an *action* verb.

Both goals and objectives may be modified as circumstances change. If the wagon train has as its goal to reach the North Platte, Nebraska, area by May 15, but mechanical failure or bad weather cause delays, then either the goal or the objectives leading to the goal will need to be modified. If an objective is to "travel seven miles a day," and so far the wagon train has averaged only five, then perhaps changing that objective to nine miles a day will help get the group back on schedule. To accomplish this, other compromises may have to be made. The group may have to start earlier and make camp later than originally planned. They may have to remove items from the wagons to lighten the load. The key point is that because both the goals and objectives they have set for themselves are specific and measurable, they are able to monitor their progress and make the necessary adjustments to accomplish their mission.

## Focused Needs Assessment

You may have noticed that the goals and objectives have been identified without conducting a needs assessment. This approach is contrary to many widely used planning methodologies that conduct a broad needs assessment as the first step in the process (Marreel & McLellan, 1998).

By first developing goals and objectives based on the direction of the organization, however, it is possible to focus the needs assessment on those things that are truly relevant. By doing so, you realize the following benefits:

- The projects identified through the information management planning process truly reflect the direction of the organization as a whole.
- You are able to make use of the considerable needs assessment work already done in the corporate planning process.
- Questionnaires and interviews can be limited to those individuals relevant to the particular goal or objective being studied.
- Unrealistic expectations developed during a broadly based needs assessment are avoided.
- The overall needs assessment process is shorter and more efficient.

Use questionnaires only as a preliminary information-gathering device. The information gathered through the questionnaires should be used as background information for the interviews. Often, the responses to the second or third follow-up interview questions produce the most useful information.

Once the interviews are complete, revisit the goals and objectives and refine them as appropriate, based on the results of the needs assessment. Goals and objectives may need to be added, deleted, or modified. In this sense, the needs assessment is a validation of the original goals and objectives.

## Strategies

A key component of an information management plan, and any plan for that matter, is the strategies. Strategies describe the framework within which you will operate. These are discussed in detail in Chapter 4.

Once you have completed the plan—that is, written an information management plan and mission statement, developed strategies, constructed measurable goals and objectives, and formulated action plans for each objective—the final requirement is to put a methodology in place to keep the information management plan relevant and current. It is fruitless to go through the considerable effort required to develop a plan, only to have it become obsolete in six months to a year due to lack of necessary ongoing review and revision.

Use the plan as an operational tool. Keep it in a three-ring binder for easy updating. Goals and objectives will be added or completed. If you have access to project planning tools, enter the plan and create Gantt charts for display and review at steering committee meetings and other venues. As circumstances change, change the plan. As new goals and objectives are introduced, add them to the plan. In this way, the plan remains current, and it will never be necessary to conduct a complete planning process again. Finally, review and renew the plan whenever the corporate plan changes. Usually this occurs at least annually (Marreel & McLellan, 1998).

# REFERENCES

Joint Commission on Accreditation of Healthcare Organizations. (1998). *Comprehensive accreditation manual for hospitals.* Oakbrook Terrance, IL: Author.

Marreel, R. D., & McLellan, J. M. (1998a). (Rev. ed.) *Information management planning workbook.* Colorado Springs, CO: RMA Publishing.

Palmer, R. P., & Varnet, H. (1990). *How to manage information: A systems approach.* Phoenix, AZ: Oryx Press.

# CHAPTER

# Strategies

It is important to understand the framework within which the information management activities will occur. At this point, we need to discuss the importance of strategies. Strategies define the framework within which your organization operates. These guidelines define how you will accomplish your goals.

Collectively, strategies represent your "game plan." Going back to the wagon train analogy, there are many examples of strategies used by those early pioneers to ensure that a journey would be as safe and uneventful as possible. First, the strategy of "strength in numbers" is obvious. This is why wagon trains were formed in the first place, so that each family would not have to make the trip on its own. A wagon train master was hired, usually someone who had prior experience with the trip. There were scouts, blacksmiths, and wheelwrights. The caravans used the strategy of following the proven route, for example, the Oregon Trail. History reports that the Donner party decided to not follow this strategy and blazed their own trail, suffering much hardship and loss of life as a result.

These were all strategies adopted by these groups to improve the odds that they would accomplish their goals and eventually achieve their mission. Strategies for accomplishing the goals of the information management plan should be developed and agreed upon in advance of, or occasionally concurrently with, the development of the plan goals and objectives.

Strategies should not be confused with goals. Strategies are the framework within which you will operate, but in and of themselves, they do not move you forward. They describe an approach of how you will proceed in specific situations. The forming of wagons into groups for mutual support and protection was a strategy, but until those wagons began moving toward specific objectives, there was no progress.

To use an information management example: "All new software application initiatives will begin with a formal needs assessment." This is a statement of a strategy. This kind of written statement gives the information management steering committee the support to say "no" to the influential person who attends a trade show and comes back with a proposal for the software application that would fix every problem in the health care organization. If statements are in place before this kind of thing happens, the committee has a much better chance of circumventing these issues without causing hurt feelings.

This very thing has happened. An organization was approached by a group of very influential neonatologists who wanted to do a study on the costs associated with treatment of pregnant women and their newborns for one year postpartum, relative to the mother's length of stay following delivery. They planned to issue a smart card to each mother. Questions arose:

- All information would have to be keyed into the smart card by office staff. Who had time for duplicate charting?
- Each office would have to have a smart card reader. Who was to pay for this?
- There were any number of entry points into the study for patients. How would results be tabulated?
- What would happen if the card was forgotten or lost?
- What if the mother went to a provider that did not have a smart card reader?
- What about laboratory and pharmacological information?

The committee asked the physicians to provide a write-up describing the project. The write-up turned out to be a statement supporting the benefits of smart card technology. The committee had become so focused on the smart card technology that the primary purpose of the study was almost secondary. Within this organization, there were better methods currently in place to gather this postpartum data, but the physicians were not interested in those. They had a solution looking for a problem.

This particular hospital had documented its information management strategies as part of its information management planning process. One of the strategies identified various input and output technologies the organization would support, and the smart card was not one of them. As a result of having that strategy written down, management was able to discuss the project with the physicians and demonstrate that the technology being proposed did not fit with the direction of the organization. The physicians accepted the decision, primarily because it was based on a larger vision of the direction of technology at this institution and had obviously been carefully evaluated and documented. Not every situation will be that successful, but at the very least, well-defined and documented strategies provide a basis for discussion.

A common strategy found in health care organizations today is, "If automation is indicated, we will buy, not build." In the early days of health care automation, there were few vendors but many programmers who could cobble a system together to automate specific tasks. But as time passed, it became evident that with more and more requests for automation, these projects were bigger than most small organizations could handle. Vendors could produce more complete packages. Although the initial cost seemed large, it proved cheaper over many years.

## TYPES OF STRATEGIES

When identifying strategies, think about problem areas within the organization. There may already be written policies and procedures in these areas. To heighten awareness and strengthen the effort, rewrite these policies and procedures as strategies.

- Infrastructure
  - System platform
  - Software platforms
  - Forms generation and approval
- Organization
  - Committees, work groups
  - Cross-functional participation
- General
  - Automation strategy
  - Process improvement strategy
  - Project prioritization
  - Standardization

## EXAMPLES OF SPECIFIC STRATEGIES

The following are some examples of specific information management strategies (Marreel & McLellan, 1998).

## Clinical Information Strategy

Information in the medical record must be timely, accurate, secure, and accessible. All information management initiatives related to clinical information will be directed toward the enhancement of these characteristics.

## Overall Automation Strategy

All information management initiatives will be solution-driven, not system-driven. For example, there is a problem in providing timely, accurate patient information to the remote health care sites. It would be desirable to have the patient information stored at the central site available at multiple remote locations. The "solution" that comes to mind is to build an "electronic medical record" and make it available over a network. This solution would involve several elements, including software applications, networks, process changes, procedural changes, and operational compromises. In order to avoid disappointments and unintended consequences, the role that a software application will or will not play in the overall solution will be clearly understood at the outset.

## Problem Assessment Strategy

Problems will be researched to identify solutions in the following order of preference:

Solutions achieved through re-engineering of existing processes, user training, and the manipulation of existing capabilities and data.

Solutions involving new software, particularly enterprisewide applications that operate on the health care organization's management hardware platform fully integrated into the existing database.

Solutions involving new departmental software applications that can operate autonomously, but be accessible on the enterprisewide local area network (LAN). Care will be taken to ensure that any systems acquired have been optimized to run over the existing network.

## Hardware/Network Strategy

Capability will be built upon and around the hardware platform selected for the health care organization's management system. To the extent possible, systems will be "open." Local area networks (LANs) will be Ethernet, supporting a standard communication protocol. A wide area network (WAN) to service remote locations will be built methodically, using dedicated lines only as network traffic warrants the cost. All system purchases will be network-enabled, with the appropriate gateways.

## System Integration Strategy

Every effort will be made to ensure that applications are integrated into a common database. To the extent that full integration is not possible or necessary, robust, real-time interfaces will be sought. For all new software applications, the required integration or interface specifications will be developed and presented to potential software vendors for feasibility and pricing. The responsibility for providing a successful interface will always fall to the vendor of choice. This will be reflected clearly in all vendor contracts.

## Input/Output Strategy

A unified approach to input/output (I/O) will be followed. The conditions under which alternate methods of entry and retrieval, other than keyboard, light pen, and printer, are appropriate will be determined by the information management steering committee. These preferred technologies would be the standards for future purchases. Before an alternate I/O method is selected for a particular application, consideration will be given to whether the technology can be used elsewhere as well.

There are several alternative I/O approaches gaining marketplace viability. These include point-of-care terminals, optical scanning, handheld devices, voice recognition, and bar code readers. Unchecked proliferation of various I/O technologies could lead to problems with training, support, and maintenance. Careful consideration will be used.

## System Support Strategy

A relatively small information technology (IT) department has been asked to support an ever-increasing number of software applications and users. In order to use the IT resources to the best advantage, a release strategy similar to that used by commercial software vendors will be implemented. Release dates will be published periodically, for example, quarterly, along with the modifications and additions that will appear in each release. In this way, system change requests can be grouped, managed, implemented, and communicated much more efficiently than if handled on a one-by-one basis.

## Information Technology Staffing

Even with the most efficient operations, staffing requirements increase as additional software applications are installed. A shortage of well-trained staff to provide support can cripple even the best of systems. Estimates of internal support requirements (IT staff training and additions) will be made for all system acquisitions and included in the estimated capital and operational costs of the system.

## Electronic Medical Record Strategy

The ability to retrieve and update the complete patient medical record electronically has long been the "holy grail" of the medical information system industry. It will remain so for many years to come; however, progress is being made with the advent of improved image capture, voice recognition, and communication capabilities.

Systems purchased today will become key components of the eventual electronic record. The manner in which a system will contribute to the realization of an electronic record will be a key consideration in the evaluation and acquisition of new systems.

## PRIORITIES

The following prioritization criteria is to be applied to each new or enhanced capability:

- Priority 1. Replace the existing applications
- Priority 2. Develop and/or improve remote-site capabilities:
  — Entry and retrieval of data on the central system
  — Communication options to and from the central site, and among remote sites
- Priority 3. Acquire and implement strategic health care organization or departmental systems
- Priority 4. Acquire and implement nonstrategic health care organization or departmental systems

Possessing agreed upon strategies, or "rules of the road," is key to the orderly conduct of any information management function. Without them, the information management steering committee will lack focus and consistency. For example, if your committee is selecting a practice management system, you would want to know the long-term direction to which the organization has agreed. It would be necessary to understand what approach will be used for processing the data. There are many options available, for example, centralized processing on a large mainframe computer, client-server processing using a standard protocol, a mini-computer system tied into a larger network, or outsourcing to a service provider. All of the considerations need to be addressed (Marreel & McLellan, 1998).

## REFERENCES

Marreel, R. D., & McLellan, J. M. (1998). (Rev. ed.). *Information management planning workbook.* Colorado Springs, CO: RMA Publishing.

# CHAPTER

# 5

# Continuum of Care

The third and final critical piece of information you should have before attempting any needs assessment is a full appreciation of your organization's continuum of care. The identity of the organization's continuum of care is something many people assume they know. These same people are often surprised when they see all services sized and documented in a form that is easily visualized, especially in today's rapidly changing health care environments.

Organizations that have historically considered themselves as inpatient acute care providers are increasing outpatient and long-term care services and decreasing inpatient care. It is easy to underestimate the extent to which technology and economics have changed the delivery of care. To do so can result in expenditures in software applications that are unwarranted, based on the direction of the organization.

For this reason, we strongly recommend that an assessment of the continuum of care be performed, as the basis for any large-scale planning effort, and that it be reviewed and updated annually. This begins the process and focuses the planning effort.

# GETTING STARTED

There are several steps to completing the continuum of care. Start by listing:

- All current services and capabilities within your health care organization
- All future services and capabilities that are planned for your organization

And then:

- Research revenue figures for each
- Analyze the size and scope of current services
- Analyze the size and scope of future services

# DRAFT AN OUTLINE

For each service, gather revenue numbers, number of episodes, estimated costs, services, and so on. Size the boxes, circles, spheres, and lines accordingly. Decide how you want to break down the information. Some possibilities are:

- By site
- By service
- By project
- By revenue
- By geographic area
- Current capabilities versus future needs

# DISPLAY YOUR CONTINUUM

Draft the overall representation and then review it with:

- Peers
- Finance
- Administration

When assessing your institution's services, it is helpful to produce a picture of what your services look like. Figure 5–1 summarizes an actual health care organization's services. When documenting your own, begin at the lowest level of detail and summarize to higher levels (Marreel & McLellan, 1998).

In Figure 5–1, "Clinics" box represents the following clinical service areas: eye, burn, wound, diabetes, hypertension, and so on. The size of each box in the diagram

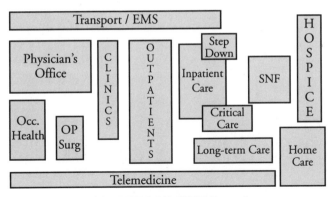

CONTINUUM OF CARE Example

**Figure 5–1** Continuum of care (Marreel & McLellan, 1998)

represents the amount of revenue generated in each service area. By assessing your services and building a picture based on revenue, the priorities for improving or adding software applications often become apparent.

Note that the continuum in Figure 5–1 reads from left to right. It moves from outpatient services to inpatient services to extended care. Telemedicine and emergency medical services (EMS) are used across the continuum.

Figure 5–2 is a worksheet that will help you organize your continuum of care. List all current services provided within each box. The subtopics running along the bottom of the figure, "Outpatient," "Inpatient," and "Extended Care," are there to assist you in thinking of longitudinal services. Work with the finance department to find revenue numbers and estimate the correct sizing of each box. Ask administration about future services that may be planned and include them in the continuum.

Use different colors, patterns, sizes, and so on to make visual impact in your continuum of care diagram. A drawing software application will make this easier. The finished continuum of care diagram should be verified and updated yearly by the information management steering committee as a part of the information management (IM) plan.

## IDENTIFY RESPONSIBLE PARTIES

After the services have been listed and sized, identify the name of the person responsible and knowledgeable for each service area. There may be several for one box, for example, in the "Clinics" box, each director's and manager's name should be listed. This comprehensive listing becomes the client database (see Figure 5–3). You will use this list to identify specific names and addresses of staff who will receive needs assessment questionnaires. These staff members will have an opportunity for input into IM decision making.

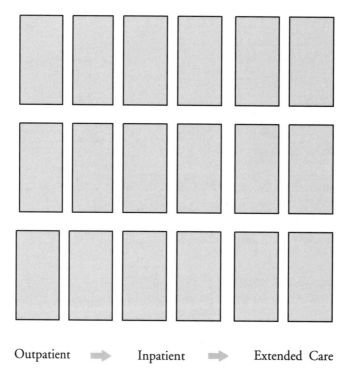

Outpatient ➡ Inpatient ➡ Extended Care

**Figure 5–2** Continuum of Care Worksheet (Marreel & McLellan, 1998)

It is important that you consider all possibilities. Develop this client list with peers to make sure that everyone with an interest in your eventual solution is included. Do not forget individuals who are external to the organization but who may be recipients of or contributors to information relevant to the project, such as state and federal regulatory agencies and third-party payers. Remember also the clients who may be involved in the future as a result of changes brought on by the project, such as the following:

- Administrative functions—accounting, finance, personnel
- Clinical functions—nursing, laboratory, radiology, pharmacy
- Clinical support functions—medical records, utilization review, quality assurance (QA)
- Providers, patients, families
- Volunteers, clergy
- Educational liaisons—students, instructors
- Payers, outside agencies, external databases

List name, title, and address of the responsible party for each service area.

Name                                    Title                                    Address

Administrative Personnel

_____

_____

_____

_____

_____

_____

_____

_____

Clinical Personnel

_____

_____

_____

_____

_____

_____

_____

Other

_____

_____

_____

_____

_____

_____

_____

_____

_____

_____

**Figure 5–3** Client database (Marreel & McLellan, 1998)

# REFERENCES

Marreel, R. D., & McLellan, J. M. (1998). (Rev. ed.). *Information management planning workbook.* Colorado Springs, CO: RMA Publishing.

# CHAPTER

# Needs Assessment

Armed with information on the direction of the organization, the information management strategies, and your continuum of care, you are finally ready to begin the needs assessment process. You should not underestimate the importance of understanding the big picture even when working on relatively small projects. Very few software applications are so small and self-contained that they do not have some impact on operations outside their immediate area. A thorough analysis is rarely a waste of time. The better the big picture is understood, the more likely the software application you select, or the modifications you propose, will effectively serve the needs of the organization.

The needs assessment activity can coincide with long-range planning, software application selection, or process revision. The level of detail depends on which of these activities the needs assessment is directed toward. The goals and objectives outlined in the information management plan were arrived at as the result of a high-level needs assessment conducted during the corporate long-range planning effort. The level of detail required to define the needs associated with a specific project is much greater. In any event, at this stage, it has normally been determined that there are *needs*. The assessment process attempts to define those needs in detail.

The following elements make up the process for preparing a needs document.

## STATEMENT OF THE PROBLEM

The problem begets the need. The problem "I am thirsty" occurs before the need "drink" is recognized. The solution will be based on availability and individual taste. It could take the form of pure water, soda, juice, tea, coffee, milk, and so on. The point is that a problem must be recognized before a need can be identified and a solution can be formulated.

You may have heard the expression, "It is a solution in search of a problem," meaning the solution is unnecessary, not needed. If the problems are clearly stated and agreed to by all concerned, unneeded solutions will be avoided, and needed solutions will be on target. There is a direct correlation between the clarity of the problem and the precision of the solution.

## STATEMENT OF THE NEED

We recognize a need based on a problem. If communication of patient information is the problem, then we look for solutions. The need is often stated in terms of a goal or objective in the information management plan. The following statement is a clear statement of a need:

> Improve the communication of outpatient information, to include individual patient demographic, financial, assessment, problem list, and treatment information for the most recent encounter, to within a three-second request/response time for all patients visiting all outpatient clinics and the ER.

The need implies the problem, but it does not propose a solution. The whole point of a needs assessment is to arrive at a solution. During the needs assessment, you evaluate the environment to arrive at a solution.

## EVALUATION OF THE CURRENT SYSTEMS

This should include both manual and automated systems that are presently used to perform the functions indicated in the statement of the problem. The evaluation consists of documenting the strengths and weaknesses of the current methods and systems: that is, "what are we currently doing well; what are we currently not doing well?"

Unless we are dealing with a totally new service or function, there is an existing way of doing things. It would be extremely rare that everything in a particular process would be "bad." Successful improvement efforts depend heavily on a thorough understanding of the strengths and weaknesses of existing processes, both manual and automated.

Resist the temptation to define all improvements in terms of systems or software applications. Sometimes tremendous improvements can be realized through training and/or modifications to existing forms and procedures.

## IDENTIFICATION OF ADDITIONAL CAPABILITIES

In addition to the things you currently do successfully, identify those things you would like to be able to do in the future. These capabilities are beyond the abilities of the systems and procedures currently in place. An extension of current capabilities may involve one or a combination of the following:

- Additions to existing systems
- Interfaces between systems or software applications
- Replacement of existing systems
- Reorganization of personnel or physical workspace
- Schedule changes
- Forms redesign
- Workflow modifications

## DOCUMENTATION OF APPLICATION NEEDS

Application needs are a combination of capabilities you currently have and do well, capabilities you currently have but do not do well, and capabilities that you do not currently have but would like to have. Collectively, they represent the solution.

Do a line-by-line description. If automation is the answer, and that is not always the case, these application capabilities can be used as a basis for a request for proposal (RFP).

## DOCUMENTATION OF OTHER NEEDS

In addition to the detailed application capabilities, if the needs assessment indicates that automation is the best alternative to meet some or all of the needs, additional non-application requirements must be identified. These may include specific hardware and software platforms, interfaces to other software applications, conversion of old files to a new format, installation assistance, future support expectations, constraints on system cost, and timing.

When looking at the overall effectiveness of the current system and assessing new software applications, use the automation strategies previously defined in the information management plan as a guide.

Prepare a needs document. This document (see Figure 6–1) is the basis for all future activities surrounding the project. It should be aimed at solving the problem that has been identified. It serves the following purposes:

- Portions may be used as a guide for process improvement activities.
- Portions may be extracted to assist in the development of an RFP and in the selection of a system.

In any event, this document should be reviewed on a regular basis. It is the checklist against which to measure success and performance of both internal and vendor activities.

## CONDUCTING A NEEDS ASSESSMENT

There is an orderly process for conducting a needs assessment. If the steps are followed chronologically and the problem is well defined initially, the resulting solution should be on target. We only need to concern ourselves thereafter with a successful implementation.

A needs assessment project has six primary sets of activities:

1. Identifying your clients
2. Developing questionnaires
3. Conducting interviews
4. Summarizing needs by client (for example, patient, provider)
5. Summarizing needs by function (for example, nursing)
6. Classifying needs in terms of:
   - Infrastructure
   - New capability
   - Modified/enhanced capability

| Capability Description | Priority |
|---|---|
| *Patient Registration:* | |
| Collect demographic data on new patients | ——— |
| Patient demographic, general clinical, and guarantor data contained on one or two screens | ——— |
| Verify demographic data on returning patients | ——— |
| Collect and verify insurance data | ——— |
| Entry and retrieval of x-ray film file number | ——— |

**Figure 6–1** Sample needs document (Marreel & McLellan, 1998)

## Identify Your Clients

In Chapter 5, we discussed the continuum of care and the importance of keeping it current. It is from the continuum of care that we identified all the potential clients or customers of information who may be affected by any given project. For each service noted in the continuum of care, individuals' names and addresses were listed on the client database worksheet. These individuals are potential recipients of the questionnaire that will be distributed during the data collection phase of the needs assessment process.

## The Questionnaire

A crucial and sometimes indispensable tool is the questionnaire. Questionnaires are used to obtain, from potential system users and beneficiaries, opinions on the strengths and weaknesses of their current processes and suggestions for improving these processes.

Questionnaires can be used at various points during the needs assessment, implementation, and follow-up process. Initially, the questionnaire is used to provide information on the environment within which the problem exists. We use the questionnaire to obtain information during steps two and three of the needs assessment process.

The questionnaire should be specific to the problem at hand, comprehensive, easy to answer, easy to evaluate, and useful to begin discussion during the follow-up interview. This is a tall order. We recommend using a focused questionnaire (see Figure 6–2). In this questionnaire, the questions remain the same, only the issue changes at the top of the form. There are five questions to answer. The respondents are given a lot of latitude. The only restriction is that their responses must apply to the problem and the need.

Filling out the form shown in Figure 6–2 does not require a large amount of time, but it does give the respondent an opportunity to think about the direction of the organization and the impact of this issue. The job of the questionnaire is to collect data. The completed questionnaire serves as a place to start discussion for a follow-up interview. By using a focused questionnaire, the questions will encourage thinking, but the responses will not get too detailed. In fact, a questionnaire that attempts to get too much detail may inhibit the results. The individuals answering the questionnaire are the "experts." Let them provide the detail. The analyst's job is to distribute the questionnaire, providing the respondent with a framework that will elicit the best results.

Figure 6–2 is an example of a generic questionnaire that is made specific by the statement of the problem and need. The respondent is asked to provide only answers that are relevant to those two things. By providing both the problem and the need, the respondent is given perspective. There should be no pride of authorship with this. The more knowledgeable the person looking at a problem, the better the solution is likely to be. Respondents may come back with, "You have the problem right, but the need is wrong."

**Needs Assessment Questionnaire**

The purpose of this assessment is to obtain your input on what is needed to effectively gather, manipulate, store, and share, data and information (Management of Information) in pursuit of a solution to the Problem and Need described below. Answer each question as thoroughly as possible. Attach additional pages if more space is required.

**Problem:** *Information required for outpatient care is often incomplete or unavailable when needed for treatment at remote clinic locations.*

**Need:** *Improve the communication of outpatient information to include individual patient demographic, financial, assessment, the problem list, and treatment information for the most recent encounter, to within a three-second request/response time for all patients visiting all outpatient clinics and the ERs.*

1. What do you perceive as the Information Management strengths in your group that will enable you to contribute to the achievement of this Need?

   _____
   _____
   _____
   _____

2. What do you perceive as the Information Management weaknesses in your group that will inhibit you from contributing to the achievement of this Need?

   _____
   _____
   _____
   _____

3. Do you perceive any physical or geographic constraints?

   _____
   _____
   _____
   _____

4. Do you perceive any organizational constraints, such as personnel, rules and regulations, procedures?

   _____
   _____
   _____
   _____

5. Summarize additional requirements not covered by the previous questions. Prioritize each in terms of High, Medium, or Low.

   _____
   _____
   _____
   _____

**Figure 6–2** Needs assessment questionnaire (Marreel & McLellan, 1998)

On the other hand, they may say, "You have the problem all wrong." Obviously, the purpose of the questionnaire is not to obtain a critique on your work; however, if this happens, think about it and discuss it. Perhaps the issue needs clarification, or maybe only part of the problem is being addressed. The respondents are the experts; they could be right.

Gather and review the completed questionnaires. Responses will vary considerably in quality and content. Some respondents will be very thorough, while others will quickly complete the questionnaire without much thought. Still others will not respond at all.

As a screening tool, questionnaires are very valuable, but they should never be used in isolation, without a follow-up interview. The questionnaire merely provides initial information that will be clarified and expanded upon in an interview setting. Some responses are sometimes misleading and need further investigation.

As an example, we were conducting an information management audit for a client with seventeen hospitals served from one data center. This organization, like others, contributed to national databases on a routine basis, with data on admissions, discharges, outcomes, number of employees, and so on. For background information, we pulled some of that data. The database reported 74 FTEs in the information systems department. After an actual head count, we came up with 123 FTEs. When questioned, the CIO admitted that he responded with the lower number so as not to be compared unfavorably with other institutions. This is not an isolated incident. It is human nature to sometimes respond to questionnaires in very self-serving ways. Both the veracity of the responses and your interpretation of them need to be validated.

## The Interview

Interviews are time-consuming. Generally, your initial session will require from forty-five minutes to an hour. Additional follow-ups may be needed. There may be twenty-five, fifty, or even more people to interview. This number will vary, of course, depending on the project. In any event, the following strategies are useful to streamline the interview process.

Since this is such a tremendous investment in time, it is helpful to prepare a checklist of the expected outcomes from each interview. This checklist will vary somewhat, depending on the individual being interviewed. For example, you would likely have different expectations for an interview with the CEO and an interview with a unit secretary. From the CEO, you would be looking for input concerning the "big picture" requirements, such as plans for additional clinics, changes in services and infrastructure, impacts on related activities, and so on. From the unit secretary, you would be more interested in a discussion of current workflow, what generates the work, specific time frames of work, data requirements, systems used, suggestions for improvement, and so on. It is all important information. The key is to collect as much information as possible on the first interview. You want to invest as little time as possible in follow-up interviews. And for certain individuals, such as the CEO, you may get only one shot.

Review and make appropriate modifications to your checklist before each interview. Include specific points from the questionnaire responses that require expansion or clarification. Forward this list to the interviewee prior to the interview so that the person can be prepared. Figure 6–3 is an example of an interview checklist.

If the number of interviews become overwhelming, you may decide to recruit some assistance. If so, you will want to ensure consistency. Role-play an interview with the interview team to demonstrate the desired approach. Review the questionnaires in advance, adding any additional key points to the interview checklist for clarification or expansion.

Conduct group interviews whenever possible. Four to six participants are a very manageable number. Form the group with individuals having a common interest relevant to the need being assessed. Whenever appropriate, include representatives from across departmental lines to obtain different perspectives. Avoid including individuals in a group who might dominate the group discussion due to either their position in the organization or their personality. These individuals should be scheduled for separate interviews.

---

**Interview Checklist**

Date: _____ Time: _____
Interviewee: _____
_____
_____
_____
_____

Interviewer: _____
  1. Get an overview of responsibilities.
  2. Get an overview of the systems used and processes followed.
  3. Identify interactions with other departments.
  4. Collect pertinent forms. (Please bring copies to the interview.)
  5. Collect relevant policies and procedures. (Please bring copies to the interview.)
  6. Validate interpretation of all questionnaire responses. Expand and clarify where necessary.
  7. In particular, clarify the answer to question number 2 on the questionnaire.
  8. Other:

---

**Figure 6–3** Interview checklist (Marreel & McLellan, 1998)

## Documenting the Results

Perhaps the most difficult task of the needs assessment process is the documentation of the interview and questionnaire results. In a needs assessment, we are concerned with identifying the required improvements or additions to procedures, systems, and workflows that will move us toward a validated solution. Knowledge of these improvements allows us to design procedures, systems, and workflows to accomplish the desired result. The terms *procedure, system,* and *workflow* are defined as follows:

- **Procedure.** A regimented routine used to perform a task
- **System.** An automated tool used to perform a task
- **Workflow.** The sequential execution of tasks that results in the completion of a unit of work

For example, a patient assessment involves a number of tasks—determining height, weight, temperature, and so on. A *procedure* is followed for each of these tasks. There are tools used to perform these procedures. One of these tools is often a *system* to record and communicate the findings of the assessment. The sequential execution of the tasks— measurement of height, weight, and temperature; documentation of findings; and so on—that results in completion of the assessment is the *workflow.*

Generally there are five types of information that come from questionnaires and interviews:

1. Unanticipated information that may affect the original definition of the problem or the need
2. A review of the current operating systems, procedures, and workflows
3. Validation of the strengths of current systems, procedures, and workflows
4. Validation of the weaknesses of current systems, procedures, and workflows
5. Suggestions for improvement to systems, procedures, and workflow toward fulfillment of the need

You will use each of these pieces of information in different ways.

## Unanticipated Information

Occasionally you will discover after talking to the "experts," the staff involved in the identified problem, that the original thesis of the needs assessment was inaccurate. Based on this new information, you will have to restate the need before proceeding further. In most cases, this may change the proposed solution, but rarely does it invalidate the work that has been done to that point. The information that has been collected will still be relevant but, at the very least, may require additional follow-up discussion in light of the new information. Restate the need, follow-up as necessary, and proceed.

## Current Systems, Procedures, and Workflow

A comprehensive understanding of current systems, procedures, and workflow is critical to successful resolution of the problem. The current way of doing things provides the foundation upon which improvements will be built. Even if old systems are totally replaced by new ones, the existing workflow will strongly influence the nature of the new system.

It is easier to comprehend this information if it is displayed visually. Therefore, organize it chronologically in a list and create a flowchart. This will help in the analysis of the situation and is useful for presentation during the walk-through, which is discussed later. This approach is easy to master and easily understood by any audience. A general overview of flowcharting is provided later in this chapter.

## Strengths of Current Systems, Procedures, and Workflows

Obviously, you do not want to overlook any of the good things that are currently being done. Any recommended solution should include these things and reinforce them, if possible. Keep this list of positives. It will be used in the walk-through and as a checklist in evaluating the proposed solution, to ensure that no strengths have been sacrificed in the process.

## Weaknesses of Current Systems, Procedures, and Workflow

This is the information that will define the core of the proposed solution. Whether it is modifications or additions to existing systems and procedures, or a complete replacement of everything, the severity and depth of existing weaknesses will determine the result.

Using your flowchart of the current process, identify the weak points and develop scenarios to correct them. Weaknesses are corrected through improved procedures, systems, or workflows. The scenarios should be based on the suggestions for improvement that were obtained during the questionnaire and interview process, and on your analysis, drawn from your own experience and knowledge.

First, construct "what-if" narratives. Process these through the flowchart. Identify the best alternatives, and come to consensus within your team. Once you are satisfied with the improved workflow, modify the flowchart to reflect the changes. The result should be one flowchart of the current workflow and a second flowchart of the revised workflow. Use the lists of strengths and weaknesses developed earlier to verify that the changes reflect all of your findings and conclusions.

## THE WALK-THROUGH

It is always prudent to validate progress from time to time during the course of a project. We derive two important benefits from this. First, we obtain valuable feedback with which to make midcourse corrections if necessary. Second, we provide valuable education to those who will be affected by the project (Marreel & McLellan, 1998).

This is accomplished through the periodic presentation of a walk-through. The purpose at this stage is to:

- Communicate the findings and recommendations of the needs assessment process to all those who were involved and will be affected by any changes
- Obtain feedback regarding the validity of the findings and appropriateness of the recommendations
- Provide information to management and users on the extent of change to functional procedures that is anticipated as a result of the new functions
- Give all concerned ample time to develop plans to accommodate the changes
- Identify issues that still need to be resolved

A walk-though generally can be accomplished in a one- to two-hour time period, depending on the scope of the project. Everyone involved in the needs assessment process should be invited. Other attendees should include clerical and administrative staff who will be using the new systems and procedures, even if they did not participate directly in the questionnaire and interview process. The more individuals you have looking at and thinking about the changes, the better the feedback will be, and the better the end product will turn out. Encourage questions and comments. It is better to have comments now than after the final changes have been put in place, when things are much more difficult to change.

The walk-though is most effective, in a large group, when projected on a screen from transparencies or directly from a laptop or personal computer. Ensure that there are enough seats for all invited. Control the temperature in the room. Concentration is difficult for two hours if the room is too hot or too cold. Take a break halfway through for ten to fifteen minutes. Keep your audience focused and involved in this experience.

Begin by stating the problem, followed by the need, for which the assessment was done. Present and discuss the flowchart that demonstrates the current workflow with existing systems and procedures. This brings the audience up to speed on what is currently done. Not everyone will be familiar with the current operation; do not assume that everyone is familiar with it. A short review provides everyone with a reference against which to evaluate the proposed changes.

Present a summary of your findings from the questionnaires and interviews. Present both the strengths and weaknesses of the current environment, and the recommendations for process improvement. Answer any questions and record comments. Add outstanding issues to the issues list. Issues lists are discussed in Chapter 9.

Next, present the flowchart of the new workflow design, reflecting changes that have been incorporated into the old environment. Describe new procedures, systems, and workflows to the best of your knowledge. Answer any questions and record comments. Add additional outstanding issues to the issues list.

The entire walk-through process should be an open forum for questions, comments, and concerns. If possible, provide handouts of the presentation and encourage attendees to review the material and provide feedback after the session. Assign a deadline for all comments to be received.

Provide feedback to the user community once all the comments have been received, evaluated, and incorporated, if appropriate, into the final design. Depending on the extent of additional changes made to the original presentation, this may take the form of an addendum to the original design or a complete rewrite. Accordingly, either distribute the changes to attendees in the mail or convene another walk-through session.

Once the new design is finalized, you are ready to proceed with the detail. Most likely, the project will involve changes to all three areas—*procedures, systems,* and *workflows.* For large projects, you may need specialists in each of these areas working in concert. For smaller projects, one or two people may do it all.

## PROCEDURES

Important or sensitive tasks that need to be performed consistently time after time are documented with a written procedure. Every organization documents procedures to some extent. Federal and state regulatory agencies require a certain level of documentation to demonstrate compliance with their operational guidelines.

In spite of this, a relatively small percentage of tasks performed in an organization are actually documented. Yet, many tasks that are impacted by a process improvement or system implementation project will be modified in some way. It is important to understand the extent and impact of procedural changes caused by new or modified expectations within the operations of an organization.

The approach to documenting these procedures should first reflect the expertise of the individuals who carry out the current functions. It is helpful to rely on an outline format to provide initial information on a particular subject. Ask several experts to simply list the tasks performed during a procedure. Sometimes, it is more effective to obtain this information directly through an interview and discussion. During the interview and discussion, take notes.

When discussing a procedure, it is most effective to sketch an outline of the tasks of the procedure, along with explanatory notes. Figure 6–4 contains procedure shorthand symbols that can be drawn freehand and applied to virtually every type of procedure. With a little practice, one can become adept at this shorthand of procedure writing.

Following the interview and discussion, the notes should be refined into the appropriate format. If the procedure is to be placed in a policy and procedure manual, then a step-by-step narrative should be written, as described in Chapter 9. If the procedure is to be described in a walk-through presentation, then the hand-drawn flowchart should be redrawn using a template. Always validate your final product with the individuals responsible for the process the procedure describes.

## WORKFLOWS

A workflow is the sequential execution of tasks that results in the completion of a unit of work. As such, a workflow is a series of one or more procedures. Workflow is documented in the same manner as procedures.

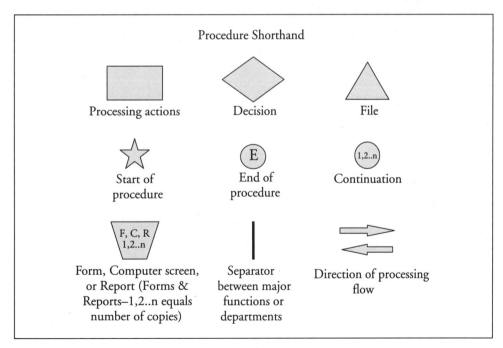

**Figure 6–4** Procedure shorthand symbols (Marreel & McLellan, 1998)

Define the unit of work that is being documented. For example, "register a new patient" is a unit of work consisting of several procedures. To complete this work, one must:

• Collect demographic and insurance data
• Enter data into the system
• Verify insurance
• Create a new chart

A different person might carry out each procedure, but the flow of the work is sequential. The data needs to be collected before it can be entered into the system and the insurance can be verified. The new chart is the last thing created. Procedures may be done in parallel with one another, but there is always a sequential flow that moves the whole process to completion.

# SYSTEMS

Many of the capabilities identified during the needs assessment likely involve automation. At this point, these needs are still defined at a high level and in very general terms. Considerably more detail must be added before these systems can be identified and purchased. If there is to be in-house development even more detail is required. Most cases will involve a combination of purchasing and in-house development.

## Interfaces

It is very rare these days for a health care organization to invest the time, personnel, and money necessary to develop its own systems. There are many health care–oriented products on the market today that satisfy the needs of health care providers. However, since there is not a truly integrated solution from any one vendor that meets all the diverse needs of a health care organization, multiple systems are often "stitched" together in order to obtain the desired functionality. Such "stitching," known as interfacing, whether done internally or by an outside vendor, requires detailed specifications. This type of detail is referred to as a program specification or, more specifically, an interface program specification.

At this point, a distinction should be made between *integrated* and *interfaced*. In an integrated system, each software application is designed to operate in a common environment. Each is complementary to, and has the same inherent access to data as, every other software application within the system. Access may be limited for security reasons to some software application functions, but if those security limitations are removed, the access is the same.

For example, suppose there is a system that consists of software functions for patient registration; billing; charting; laboratory specimen collection, processing, and reporting; medication requests; order management; and inventory control. The system is integrated if each of the functions can be accessed through a common user entry point, and the user is able to display, update, and manipulate data entered through any function, without either sending data or requesting data directly to or from another function. So, if all the data collected and stored during a patient registration process can be immediately accessed from that storage location for use by every other function, and the user can move between patient registration and order management without reidentifying herself to the new function, the system is said to be integrated.

Systems are *interfaced,* if it is necessary for one software application to send data to another software application before the first application can access it. So, if patient registration data is stored on the patient registration database and also electronically sent to the laboratory system for storage on the laboratory system database, those systems are said to be interfaced.

Another example would be the difference between a train and a bus. A train consists of multiple cars designed for varying purposes, hooked together to form the whole train. The engineer, passenger, baggage, and eating facilities are located in separate vehicles. A train is a collection of interfaces, or an interfaced system. A bus, however, is one unit, containing driver, passenger, baggage, and eating facilities. There is only one vehicle. It is easy to move from one area to the others. A bus is an integrated system.

Much is written in the literature and by the vendor community about the desirability of fully integrated systems. Integration has become a marketing tool used by vendors to differentiate themselves in the health care marketplace. The fact is, one fully integrated system, able to meet all the software application needs of a modern health care organization, is still a pipe dream, a marketer's hyperbole. No one is able to offer more than partial integration. Therefore, at this time, your systems will be a combination of integrated and interfaced software applications.

In spite of the rhetoric, this might not be all bad. Is it possible that too much emphasis is placed on integration? As in the example of the train, there are certain advantages to interfaced systems. There is certainly great flexibility; cars for specialized purposes can be added or removed, depending on need. Changes to the design of specialized cars can be made without affecting the rest of the system. Such changes are certainly more economical than they would be in the fully integrated bus.

Standardization is the key. The train is a successful mode of transportation because of standardization. The train cars are designed to be interfaced to one another with standardized couplers, track gauge, and carriages. System integration is an issue because software applications are not currently designed with standardization in mind. Each vendor is defining its own standards, making interfaces difficult, cumbersome, and inefficient as a result.

Efforts have been made to develop a common interface standard. Health Level Seven (HL7) is a group attempting to establish standards within health care organizations for the electronic exchange of text messages, including data on admissions, discharges, transfers, financial transactions, scheduling, and nursing management. The initial standards are a work in progress that all of today's vendors say they support, but these standards are often circumvented in practice by the vendor's proprietary interface.

## Detail Specifications

Detailed specifications, whether used for system selection or program development, evolve from the needs assessment. Specifications are developed in layers (see Figure 6–5). The very highest specification layer is at the information management planning level that was discussed previously. It is represented by the information management goals and objectives identified in the plan.

The next layer contains the application and infrastructure requirements developed as the result of the needs assessment that is conducted for a particular objective in the information management plan. If the software application is to be acquired from a vendor, or if an existing system is to be reinstalled, this is the lowest level of detail required.

Figure 6–6 is an example of detailed requirements at this level. These requirements may include specific hardware platforms, data input/output technologies, network technologies, hardware capacity and expandability, operating system specifications, functional characteristics of the software applications, and available interfaces to other systems.

**Specification Development Process**

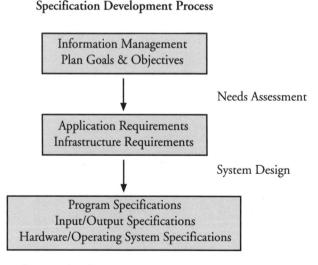

**Figure 6–5** Specification development process

| Capability Description |
|---|
| Multiuser system expandable to _____ number workstations at multiple sites. |
| Individual security by function. |
| Standard operating system used by major vendors. |
| Standard application programming language used by major vendors. |
| On-line access to all data with a high-level report writer. |
| User-defined purge parameters including: |
|    Patient/account demographic files. |
|    Patient/account transaction files. |
| PC file transfer capability (upload/download). |

**Figure 6–6** Detailed requirements

For a software application system selection, these detailed requirements are organized into a formal document called a request for proposal (RFP). The RFP is sent to software application vendors known to sell the applications requested in the proposal. The RFP is discussed in detail in Chapter 7.

The final layer of detail is the level from which software programmers develop software application programs. Unless you work in an organization that develops its own applications, you may never need to get to this level. There are instances, however, when detailed specifications are required even when software applications are acquired from a vendor. Two of the most common occurrences are for the development of interface specifications and for the development of input/output specifications.

## Interface Specifications

Often when a software application is purchased, there is a desire to connect the new system to one or more existing systems so that useful data can be exchanged between systems. A common example is an admission, discharge, and transfer system interfaced to a laboratory system. Interface specifications need to be written to define the interface. The interface specifications describe five things:

1. The data to be passed
2. The format of the record containing the data to be passed
3. The direction of the interface, one-way or bidirectional
4. The communication protocol
5. What is to happen in the event of an error

The data to be passed is formatted into a record consisting of one or more data elements, or fields. A data element is the smallest piece of useable information in the record. For example, in a record containing patient demographic data, a list of typical data elements might be: patient number, patient's first name, patient's middle initial, patient's last name, date of birth, sex, marital status, street address, phone, city, state, and zip code. The interface specifications would contain detail on the length of each field, the type of data in each field (numeric, alphanumeric, floating point), conditions under which each field should be included in or excluded from the record, editing criteria, and any manipulation of the data element that must be done before it is included in the record.

The format of the record is described by the data elements and the sequence in which the data elements are to appear in the record. There can be many types of records. One record may contain patient demographic data, another may contain financial data, and another may contain patient assessment data.

The first record in a series of records is often a specialized record called a *header record,* and the last record in a series is often a specialized record called a *footer record.* The header record is sent first. It signals to the receiving program that records containing data are being sent. The receiving program, upon analyzing the header record, branches to the appropriate part of the program to process the incoming records. The actions of the receiving program may vary depending upon the information it receives in the header record.

The function of the footer record is quite simple. It signals to the receiving program that there are no more records to be sent. Header and footer records are also useful for detecting transmission errors. If the footer record has a field indicating the number of records that were sent, say ten, and only nine were received, then the receiving program would detect an error, and appropriate measures would be taken. These are called error-handling procedures.

Data can be passed in either direction across an interface between two systems. One-way communication is less complex than bidirectional communication, but the data formatting and record handling concepts are the same.

A communication protocol is a description of the process that will be used to establish communication between systems. For example, if I were to tell you in advance that when, and only when, I tap you on the left shoulder, you are to drop whatever you are doing and listen, because I will have something important to say, that would be our communication protocol. If I cleared my throat or tapped you on the arm, you would act as if I was not even there.

Essentially a communication protocol is a tap on the shoulder by the sending program to the receiving program. The sending program expects a response from the receiving program, indicating that it is ready to receive whatever data is to be sent, in much the same way as you would visually communicate to me that I had your attention as soon as you felt the tap on your shoulder.

Communication protocol will be determined based on the computing infrastructure at your organization. Your own systems people or the vendor will likely know what it should be.

## Input/Output Specifications

### Input Specifications

Virtually all applications are developed for the purpose of manipulating data that are given to them. That manipulation may result in the data being stored in a file, sent to another program for further manipulation, displayed on a monitor, or printed in a report. In the same way that the characteristics and format of data are defined in the interface specification previously discussed, the characteristics and format of input and output data must be defined.

Input specifications describe the characteristics and layout of data to be entered into the system. These specifications contain detail on the length of each field, the type of data in each field (numeric, alphanumeric, floating point), conditions under which each field should be included in or excluded from the record, editing criteria, default values, dependencies on the contents of other fields, and the position of the field on the screen or form.

Input specifications are most often developed for either paper data collection forms or screen layouts. The screen is laid out much like a paper form would be designed. The design is reflective of the medium. A paper form may be laid out in an 8.5" by 11" format, whereas a screen design form may be in an 80 character by 20 lines format. In any event, the object is the same—to provide a vehicle with which to collect all the desired data in the most effective and efficient manner possible.

Input specifications must be developed for whatever means will be used to enter the data. In addition to forms and screens, input specifications are also needed for bar code readers, voice entry, instrumentation interfaces, and handheld devices.

### Output Specifications

Output specifications are conceptually the same as input specifications, only in reverse. The purpose is to present data that has been manipulated or stored by a software application in a format that is the most useful. To do so, the same data may be presented in several different ways, depending upon how it will be used. In most instances, we do not want to present just a stream of data; we want to present useful information. Laboratory results from a chemistry profile are just data. Only when those results become associated with a particular patient do they become useful information.

The most common types of output specifications are report and screen specifications. The key characteristics are:

- The length of each field
- The type of data in each field
- Conditions under which each field should be included in or excluded from the output
- Default values
- Dependencies on the contents of other fields
- The position of the field on the screen or report

Unless you are involved in a system development project, the three types of specifications we have discussed—interface, input, and output—are the only ones you will likely be involved in developing. Purchased systems are relatively generic, and it is quite common to need modifications to screens and reports to better meet the specific needs of individual organizations. Some vendors provide tools to allow customers to make these changes themselves. In other cases, once the specifications are developed, the vendor's programming staff makes the changes.

## DATA ORGANIZATION

Data are the smallest units of information that we store, retrieve, and/or edit. Data is typically organized into groups or categories. All data must be organized in a logical structure so that it can be labeled, indexed, and easily located for retrieval. Each group is more complex than the one before (Saba & McCormick, 1995):

- **Character.** A single letter or number or special character such as a punctuation mark
- **Field.** Contains a set of related characters, for example, a patient name, John Smith
- **Record.** A collection of related fields, for example, John Smith's admission data. There may be several fields, for example, name, address, age, sex, phone number, medical number, all forming a record.
- **File.** A collection of related records. All the patients in the hospital on January 15th could form a file. There are several different kinds of files, including:
  - **Master File.** A complete file containing all permanent records up to the last update
  - **Transaction or Update File.** Contains recent changes to records that will be used to update the master file
  - **Report or Sort Files.** Temporary files used to generate a report or display

• **Database.** The highest level of storage. It consists of groups of related files. It is an organized collection. Databases are usually managed by software designed specifically for this purpose called database management systems (DBMS).

## DATABASES

There are several types of database structures that are commonly used:

• Hierarchical database
• Network database
• Relational database

## Hierarchical Database

In a hierarchical database (see Figure 6–7), fields or records are structured like a tree. Data are arranged by order of rank, with all data connected to the same base or root. This structure is common to mainframes and minicomputer systems (O'Leary & O'Leary, 1997).

There are issues with the hierarchical structure. If one of the data elements is deleted, the elements that are attached to it are deleted as well. Even more significant is the limitation caused by the rigid structure and the absence of connections between the branches. Like the limbs of a tree, if a limb is cut, all the branches emanating from the

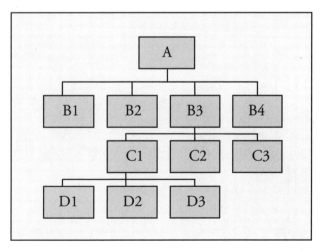

**Figure 6–7** Example of a hierarchical database
In order to access data element D3, the database access system must take the path A → B3 → C1 → D3. This arrangement is very inefficient when dealing with many data requests in a large complex database.

limb are cut too. Each addition or modification of a data element within the hierarchy requires a reorganization of the database. Since the data elements, like the tree, are all connected to the main trunk, access to those elements can be made only through the trunk, and data elements can only be defined relative to the hierarchy, not to each other. Such an approach is inefficient, since there is no direct accessibility to individual elements.

## Network Database

The network database (see Figure 6–8) also has a hierarchical arrangement. However, every branch may be connected to more than one level. This is called a "many-to-many" relationship. There are additional connections, called pointers, that link the branches due to some type of relationship, such as a patient name, physician name, or diagnosis. The selection of variables to be linked together influences the structure of the database and the way the database is accessed.

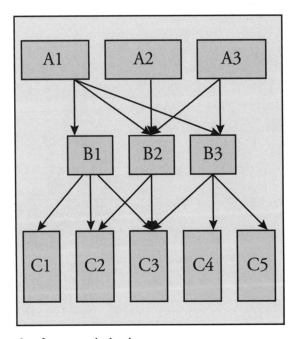

**Figure 6–8** Example of a network database
Data element C3 can be accessed through A1, A2, or A3. The network database delivers improved efficiency, but retains the rigid inflexibility of the hierarchical database.

## Relational Database

The most flexible type of organization is the relational database (see Figure 6–9). In this structure, there are no access paths down a hierarchy to an item of data. Rather, the data elements are stored in different tables, each of which consists of rows and columns. The most valuable feature of a relational database is the simplicity. Entries can be easily added, deleted, and modified.

## Available Databases

Databases help users stay current and plan. Among the hundreds of databases available to help users with both general and specific business purposes are the following (O'Leary & O'Leary, 1997):

• Business directories providing addresses, financial and marketing information, products, and trade and brand names

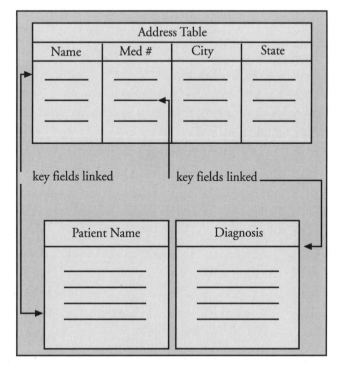

**Figure 6–9** Example of a relational database
The relational database offers relative efficiency and can be modified without affecting the rest of the database.

- Demographic data, such as county and city statistics, current estimates on population and income, employment statistics, census data, and so on
- Business statistical information, such as financial information on publicly traded companies, market potential of certain retail stores, and other business data and information
- Text databases providing articles from business publications, press releases, reviews on companies and products, and so on

## Database Security

Security of a database is a vital issue. There is concern that data stored on databases will be used for the wrong purposes or that unauthorized users will gain access to a database. Safeguards must be in place and constantly monitored.

## REFERENCES

Marreel, R. D., & McLellan, J. M. (1998a). (Rev. ed.). *Information management planning workbook.* Colorado Springs, CO: RMA Publishing.

Marreel, R. D., & McLellan, J. M. (1998b) (Rev. ed.). *JCAHO I.M. survey preparation workbook.* Colorado Springs, CO: RMA Publishing.

O'Leary, T. J., & O'Leary, L. I. (1997). *Computing essentials.* New York: McGraw-Hill.

Saba, V. K., & McCormick, K. A. (1995). *Essentials of computers for nurses.* New York: McGraw-Hill.

# CHAPTER

# System Selection

## ORGANIZING THE EFFORT

Once the needs assessment is complete, you are ready to begin selection of a software application or system. For the purposes of this chapter and the remainder of the text, it will be assumed that the application software identified by the needs assessment will be purchased from a vendor, rather than developed in-house. It is extremely rare for a health care organization to develop its own application software these days. The effort is just too expensive and time-consuming. It is much more likely that a suitable product will be purchased from a vendor and then modified, using tools provided by the vendor, to meet specific needs of the organization.

It is important to organize the system selection effort in advance—to lay out a schedule and outline the major milestones to be accomplished. Figure 7–1 is an example of a schedule with corresponding responsibilities for selection of a major health information system (HIS). The schedule in this instance outlines an eleven-month process. The schedule would be shortened for smaller systems. It is really a best-case scenario. There is any number of places where this schedule could expand. It is best, however, to

| System Selection Schedule | | |
|---|---|---|
| **Agenda** | **Responsible Party** | **Dates** |
| Develop a Request for Information (RFI) | Selection Committee | 1/15 to 2/1 |
| Send to selected vendors | Selection Committee | 2/4 |
| Develop the Request for Proposal (RFP) | Selection Committee | 1/15 to 3/14 |
| RFI responses due | Vendors | 3/5 |
| Evaluate RFIs | Selection Committee | 3/5 to 3/10 |
| Present findings | Selection Committee | 3/12 |
| Forward RFP to selected vendors | Selection Committee | 3/15 |
| RFP responses due | Vendors | 5/1 |
| Evaluate RFPs | Selection Committee | 5/1 to 5/21 |
| Present semifinalists | Selection Committee | 5/25 |
| Prepare for on-site system demonstrations | Selection Committee | 5/26 to 6/1 |
| On-site system demonstrations | Vendors | 6/15 to 7/1 |
| Present findings | Selection Committee | 7/10 |
| Prepare for site visits | Sel Committee/Vendors | 7/11 |
| Conduct site visits | Sel Committee/Vendors | 8/1 to 8/14 |
| Present recommended vendor-of-choice | Selection Committee | 8/25 |
| Negotiate the contract | Administration/Vendor | 9/15 to 10/15 |
| Begin implementation | Impl Workgroup/Vendor | 11/15 |

**Figure 7–1** System selection schedule

develop a reasonable schedule, rather than to include too much padding. A tight schedule is more likely to keep everyone focused. Adjustments will likely be required anyway, regardless of how much, or how little, padding is included initially.

Review the schedule with the information management steering committee. It is important to have consensus on both responsibilities and time frames, since some activities, such as site visits, can demand significant blocks of time from the participants. It is better to work out as many scheduling conflicts as possible early in the process.

The goal of the system selection process is to find the product and vendor with the combined characteristics that most closely fit the needs of the organization. The characteristics of both the product and the vendor are important. Too often, all of the attention is given to the product. The shortcomings of the vendor, from poor implementation support to ineffectual product support after implementation, are sometimes overlooked. Stories abound of great products that were never properly implemented because of poor follow-through by the vendor.

There are also too many instances when a product is purchased because the buyer "fell in love" with the vendor, not the product. In other instances, buyers have paid, and continued paying through annual fees, far too much for the functionality and services they received. These pitfalls can be avoided. To do so, the system selection process should:

- Be approached with objectivity throughout the process
- Assess the strengths and weaknesses of the *product* relative to the organization's needs
- Assess the strengths and weaknesses of the *vendor* relative to the organization's needs
- Assess the value of the products and services

## OBJECTIVITY

As with any major purchase, it is best to do a little research beforehand. You want to keep the persuasive powers of the salesperson out of the purchase decision for as long as possible. At some point, you will have to confront the vendor and listen to all the reasons why you should select its product over the others. This is valuable input, but only after a lot of preparation on your part.

Initially, the information balance is in the favor of the vendors. The salespeople have the most knowledge. They understand the strengths and weaknesses of their products. They have a good understanding of the health care industry needs, since that is the industry they serve. Moreover, based on dealings with prior prospects, they can anticipate many of the questions and concerns that you may raise. Before you talk with vendors, you need to alter the information balance in your favor.

If you were in the market for a new car, you would probably try to find out as much as possible about what is available and what is right for your needs before you began negotiating with the salesperson at the dealership. A smooth-talking salesperson can turn even the most sophisticated buyer's brain to mush. Rationality takes a holiday, causing the buyer to drive away with the biggest model, with all the options—including the built-in speakerphone and navigation system, even though the buyer may live alone, rarely get phone calls, and only use the car to drive to work and back.

Altering the information balance takes preparation and self-control. In a system selection process, preparation is accomplished with a thorough needs assessment, followed by a well-constructed request for proposal (RFP) and RFP evaluation process. Self-control is maintained through effective organization and leadership of the system selection process.

## ORGANIZATION

System selection falls under the direction of the information management steering committee. Since the steering committee has responsibility over a broad agenda, it is not normally the appropriate group to carry out all the detailed tasks involved in system selection. The actual system selection should be viewed as one more project under the information management steering committee's oversight. A project work group should be formed known as the system selection committee. This group has direct responsibility for carrying out the detailed activities involved in selection of the system.

The system selection committee reportd to, and consults with, the steering committee for guidance throughout the selection process. It is generally composed of an interdisciplinary group, including individuals with expertise in informatics to shepherd the group through the process, and individuals with specific knowledge of the functional environment within which the applications will operate.

As with the needs assessment process, the continuum of care document should be consulted to ensure that all the appropriate functional areas are represented. The selection committee should not be so large, however, that it becomes an obstacle to progress. Try to achieve an equal balance. For an HIS, the selection group should include representatives from across the continuum of care. For departmental systems, the representation would be more localized.

# REQUEST FOR INFORMATION VERSUS REQUEST FOR PROPOSAL

## Request for Information (RFI)

The purpose of the Request for Information (RFI) is to determine which vendors and products are appropriate for investigation. It is used as a tool to screen vendors before they are sent a request for proposal (RFP). The RFI contains general information about your organization, the current operational environment in which the future system will be implemented, the technical environment, and the primary capabilities you are looking for in this specific software application. The vendor is asked to describe how its products and services fit this environment. Figure 7–2 outlines the typical contents of an RFI.

It is a good idea to define your expectations in regard to the format of the response; otherwise, you will be faced with sorting through stacks of glossy marketing material in order to pull the information you are looking for. In the example in Figure 7–2, the vendors are asked to confine their comments to one page per product or service being described. Marketing material is to be separate from these one-page descriptions. If they honor this request, and that is not a given, reviewing the responses will be much easier and less time-consuming for your organization.

Sometimes an RFI, prior to sending out an RFP, is warranted, but not always. This is really a judgment call, based on the comfort level of the selection committee with their current level of knowledge of the vendors marketing the applications of interest. You may be aware of ten vendors offering systems with the same applications. A complete RFP process that includes that many vendors would be very time-consuming, so it is in your interest to quickly eliminate those who are clearly not good candidates.

---

### Example RFI

**Purpose**

The purpose of this document is to obtain information on available Information Management systems that could be used to meet the current and future needs of General Hospital (GH). Responses to this Request for Information (RFI) will be used as a basis for selecting vendors to receive a Request for Proposal (RFP) for further evaluation, eventually leading to the acquisition and implementation of an Information Management system. A total of ten vendors are receiving this solicitation.

**General Background**

General Hospital (GH) is a multifacility acute care organization with headquarters in Chicago. There is a total of seventeen hospitals located in Illinois, Indiana, and Wisconsin. Services include Acute Care, Intensive Care, Inpatient/Outpatient Surgery, Emergency Medicine, Multispecialty Outpatient Clinics, Home Health, and Skilled Nursing Care served from a central processing facility.

**Current Operating Environment**

GH is growing in terms of number and size of facilities, and services offered. In order to meet its ever-increasing need for information, GH is in the process of upgrading, adding to, and replacing a number of its current systems. GH's ultimate goal is to have a fully integrated system able to meet the needs of Inpatient, Outpatient, and Extended Care; Financial Management; Managed Care; and Executive Information.

**Technical Environment**

Several computer systems are currently being used to meet GH's need for automation. These systems include: an internally developed PCS-based HIS system for Patient Management, Orders, Results and Charting, SMS shared financial systems for Patient Billing, AR and Collections; Accounts Payable, General Ledger, Payroll and Personnel. There are multiple stand-alone systems including Lab, Pharmacy, Cost Accounting, and Executive Decision Support. Applications are run on a mixture of mainframe, minicomputer, and microcomputer platforms. The mainframe is an IBM 3090 MVS. The minicomputers are primarily DEC and IBM. Microsoft NT is the client/server environment of choice.

**Required Features**

Due to the increased complexity of required capabilities, GH needs to replace several existing applications and add new ones with an integrated system that is less costly and time-consuming to maintain.

Replace current Patient Management, Orders, Results and Charting, Patient Billing, AR and Collections; Accounts Payable, General Ledger Accounts Payable systems.

Add managed care Enrollment, Eligibility, Referral Management, and Administrative Reporting; Outcomes Management, Outpatient Management, and Physician Practice Management systems.

Add Data Warehousing and Decision Support systems.

Upgrade existing hardware and network platforms.

It is understood that a single vendor may not be able to provide every application listed above.

---

**Figure 7–2** Example RFI

The system must demonstrate the ability to expand in a building-block approach, as sites and services are added and volume increases, without the need to replace existing hardware or software.

If you believe the products and services you provide qualify as candidates to meet the above requirements, please forward information on the products, the number of installations for each product, and the hardware and operating platform required. Please limit your responses to a maximum of one page per product or service. Any preprinted marketing material you wish to send must be segregated from the one-page responses. The deadline for response is [date]. Please direct responses and all inquiries to:

R. D. Smith
PO Box 123
Chicago, IL 60614    (555) 555-1212

**Figure 7–2** (continued)

Circumstances vary, of course, but your goal in most cases should be to reduce the number of vendors who receive the RFP to no more than five. If you can do this without the RFI, go for it.

## Request for Proposal (RFP)

Because of the general nature of the RFI, the RFI is not a substitute for an RFP. As we will see later, the detailed responses to an RFP are critical to a successful selection and implementation process.

The RFP is a tool used to select the vendor, products, and services to be purchased. It recites in detail the needs of the buyer in such a way that the buyer can compare several vendors to arrive at the best solution for the organization. Since presumably all the vendors receiving the RFP offer the applications of interest, the detail is crucial to the task of differentiating them from one another.

There are many possible formats for an RFP. The one we have found to be very effective contains the following eight sections:

1. Introduction
2. Background information
3. Future automation requirements
4. General requirements for bidding
5. System capability requirements
6. Hardware and system software
7. Vendor support
8. System costs

### *Introduction and Background Information*

If an RFI was produced prior to the RFP, the first two sections of the RFP document will contain the same kind of background information that was provided in the first four sections of the RFI, only in expanded form. In Figure 7–3, notice the introduction is virtually the same as in the RFI in Figure 7–2. There is nothing to be added.

In the background section, however, the RFP should include detail relevant to the software applications of interest. The detail should correspond to the scope of the application. As appropriate, include such things as the number of beds, number of outpatient visits, current number of relevant transactions (for example, orders processed), geographic location of facilities to be served, size of existing computer network, number of terminals, number and type of users served, and so on.

Figure 7–4 is a template for the background section of a clinic management and managed care system RFP. The same level of detail appropriate to the applications of interest should be provided in any RFP.

### *Future Automation Requirements*

Future confusion and misunderstanding can be avoided by providing good information to the vendors up front in these sections. Such information enables them to make a response that is appropriate to the size and scope of your environment. Once your selection is made, you will expect the vendor to stand behind the product and the representations made during the sale. The vendor can only be expected to do this if adequate detailed information about your business and future plans is available to the vendor.

---

**RFP INTRODUCTION**

The purpose of this document is to obtain information on available Clinic Management and Managed Care Systems that could be used to meet the current and future needs of [enter your practice name here]. Responses to this Request for Proposal will be used as a basis for selecting vendors for further evaluation, eventually leading to the acquisition and implementation of a Clinic Management and Managed Care System. [Enter number of vendors being solicited] vendors are receiving this solicitation.

We request that your response *arrive* at the address listed below no later than [time], [date], [year]. We intend to notify those vendors selected for further consideration by [date], [year].

Direct all inquiries and correspondence to:
Enter the Name
Address
Telephone and fax numbers of the individual responsible for the responses.

---

**Figure 7–3** RFP introduction, RMA advantages

**BACKGROUND INFORMATION**

[Enter a description of the environment here.]

*It is important to clearly describe the nature of the practice. Include the number of physicians and other providers; the specialties represented; in-house services such as lab or radiology; any affiliations with provider networks or other heath care organizations; expected growth over the next five years in terms of new services, additional providers, new affiliations; and so on. Future confusion and misunderstanding can be avoided by providing good information to the vendors in this section. Such information enables them to make a response that is appropriate to the size and scope of your practice. Once your selection is made you will expect the vendor to stand behind the product and the representations made during the sale. The vendor can only be expected to do this if adequate detailed information about your business and future plans is available to the vendor.*

The practice gross revenue is derived from:

Fee for Service _____%
Managed Care _____%
Medicare _____%
Public Aid _____%

*If you are replacing an existing system, provide a description of the current system.*

[Enter your practice name here] wishes to replace/enhance its current software for the following applications:

[Enter your current applications here, for example:

    Patient Registration
    Accounts Receivable
    Collections
    Claims Processing
    Third-party Management
    Appointment Scheduling
    Productivity Reporting.]

These applications run on the following hardware:
[Enter your current hardware configuration here.]
Current volumes include:
Average number of visits per week by location:

    Main location _____
    Other location _____

Number of patients in the current system: _____
Number of accounts in the current system: _____
Number of active accounts in the current system: _____
Number of data entry transactions per month: _____
Number of collection letters per month: _____
Number of statements per month: _____
Number of physicians, etc., to bill for: _____
Number of insurance claims per month: _____

**Figure 7–4** Background information

## General Requirements for Bidding

The fourth section, general requirements for bidding, outlines the rules the vendors are to follow in responding to the RFP. These rules may be common to the way your organization wants to do business and are therefore based on current practices followed by your purchasing department. Figure 7–5 is an example of a typical fourth section in an RFP.

## System Capability Requirements

It is to your benefit to develop a highly structured format in this section of the RFP. The structure places constraints on responses, which allows a one-to-one comparison between vendors. An objective comparison can only be made if the responses are framed the same way, regardless of who is answering the question. In scholastic terms, we are giving the vendor a true/false and a multiple-choice test, not an essay test.

The format we recommend is one we call the *"yes, no, maybe so"* format. The vendor is asked to respond to a series of detailed capabilities, in regard to whether each capability is, within the vendor's proposed system, *available, not available, or not available but willing to provide.*

Figures 7–6 and 7–7 are examples of the general systems requirements and the specific system requirements for a clinic management and managed care system formatted this way. The specific system requirements can be quite lengthy, depending on the applications of interest. The requirement section of the RFP that is used for this example continues for fifty-eight pages. The applications include patient registration, scheduling, order entry, medical records, accounts receivable, collections, managed care payment processing, contract/benefit plan, reinsurance, enrollment, referral processing, claims adjudication, coordination of benefits, utilization review/quality assurance, and management reporting.

Creation of a document of this magnitude can be a daunting task. There are ways to make it easier. Requests for proposals can be purchased from a company that publishes generic RFPs for the applications of interest. In addition, they may be obtained through contacts at professional associations or neighboring hospitals. Finally, the outline of the system requirements section can be developed from vendor literature describing system features and functions, which can be obtained either through the RFI or directly on request from the vendor. Any of these provide a baseline. Share them with your users, and customize them to fit your specific needs.

Whatever the method, resist the temptation to shortcut this portion of the RFP. Your diligence will be rewarded with a better selection, a better contract, and a better implementation.

## Hardware and System Software

In the hardware and system software section, the sixth section, the vendor is expected to specify the configuration of equipment and operating system software required to

## GENERAL REQUIREMENTS FOR BIDDING

The following are the general requirements for bidding. These requirements should be followed by all vendors submitting a bid. Failure to do so may result in your exclusion from further consideration.

**Delivery of bid:** The original and two copies of the bid document must be received in the office of R. D. Smith no later than [date], [year].

**Bid format:** All bids must be in the format requested.

**Price guarantee:** All prices shall be effective for at least six months following the date of the proposal. The vendor will warrant that the prices quoted are all inclusive; covering hardware, software, implementation, and training expenses, required to successfully install and operate the proposed system. The vendor shall further warrant that there are no hidden costs, which may surface following final acceptance. Any exceptions to this should be specifically stated. We reserve the right to purchase the hardware from another source; therefore, the software and hardware prices must be quoted separately.

**Changes in bid before closing date:** Any changes before the closing date must be made in writing. These changes should be sent to the attention of R. D. Smith, and received no later than [date], [year].

**Changes in bid after closing date:** The bid will not be subject to change after the closing date.

**Withdrawal of bid before closing date:** The vendor may withdraw the bid at any time.

**Standard contract:** The vendor shall include one copy of its standard contract with the bid submission.

**Bid expense:** The vendor will be responsible for any and all expenses associated with the preparation of this bid.

**Modification of bid:** We reserve the right to consider bids, or modifications to the bid, received after the date indicated, but before a vendor is selected, should such action be in the best interest of General Hospital.

**Clarification of the RFP:** Any explanation desired by the vendor regarding the meaning or interpretation of the RFP must be requested in writing and in sufficient time for a reply to the request. Any interpretation made will be in the form of a letter, which will also be furnished to all recipients of this RFP. Oral interpretations or explanations will not be provided.

**RFP as part of contract:** Vendor must agree that the vendor's response to this RFP and subsequent representations or clarifications regarding the proposal shall be included in the final contract.

**Delivery and installation:** All prices for equipment will include installation in a manner that is acceptable to General Hospital, and will be F.O.B. destination.

**Vendor viability:** General Hospital will expect the vendor to furnish supplementary information on the financial status of the vendor.

**Software guarantee:** The vendor must guarantee that the application software described in the response to the RFP will be delivered free of errors and will function as indicated.

**Figure 7–5** General requirements for bidding

---

**Contract negotiations:** General Hospital reserves the right to negotiate with one or more vendors in order to arrive at a final selection.

**Contact of vendor clients:** General Hospital reserves the right to contact by telephone, or arrange a visit to, any or all of the vendor's client references. Contacts may be made without the assistance of the vendor.

**On-site demonstrations:** The vendor will be expected to provide, at General Hospital's request, on-site demonstrations of the vendor's system. This should be done through the use of terminals and printers operating in a live or simulated live mode.

**Documentation:** The vendor will provide, at General Hospital's request, examples of its documentation for the installation, training, and operation associated with its system.

---

**Figure 7–5** (continued)

run the software application. It should be made very clear that the vendor is expected to propose a configuration that will meet the performance and transaction requirements outlined in the RFP. Too often, in order to be competitive, a vendor will propose under-sized hardware components to keep the price down. This is not a basis for a fair comparison. Only the vendor is in a position to determine the appropriate hardware configuration.

The vendor's estimate is based on experience at other installations and performance tests under various configurations, transaction types, and volumes. Such tests are called benchmarks. If accurate data has been provided in the background section concerning projected transaction volumes and locations and number of system users, the vendor should be able to estimate the appropriate sizing for the system.

It should be made clear in the RFP, and in subsequent conversations with the vendor, that if the vendor is selected, the vendor is responsible for any configuration upgrades required to meet the performance criteria set forth in the RFP. In order to enforce this, you must be able to demonstrate that the data you provided are accurate. A significant increase in transactions or users would, of course, relieve the vendor of its obligation. Figure 7–8 displays the main elements of the sixth section of the RFP. Additional items that the vendor should be asked to respond to are:

- Recommended parts inventory to keep on hand for each piece of hardware described
- A description of the operating environment required for the proposed system, including power, air conditioning, recommended UPS capacity, and physical environmental requirements, for example, raised floor, humidity and temperature ranges
- Estimated square footage for the main computer room, if required, to house the equipment

| GENERAL SYSTEM CAPABILITIES | | | | |
|---|---|---|---|---|
| Please indicate whether or not you would be able to provide the capability listed below. Indicate your response with an "X" in the columns provided. | | | | |
| Capability Description | Currently available | Not available but willing to provide | Not available, not willing to provide | Comments |
| Multiuser system expandable to ___ number workstations at multiple sites | | | | |
| Individual security by function | | | | |
| Standard operating system used by major vendors | | | | |
| Application programming language used by others | | | | |
| On-line access to all data with a high-level report writer | | | | |
| User-defined purge parameters including: | | | | |
| Patient/account demographic files | | | | |
| Patient/account transaction files | | | | |
| Ability to use PCs as terminals | | | | |
| Standard off-the-shelf hardware components from a major vendor | | | | |
| Local support for both hardware and software | | | | |
| Ability to limit access to patient information at various levels: | | | | |
| Access to the Patient Index by all physicians at all locations | | | | |
| Access to detailed patient data limited by physician or group of physicians | | | | |
| Access to schedule data by all physicians at all locations | | | | |
| Access to detailed patient data limited by physician or group of physicians | | | | |
| Proven performance record for both hardware and software | | | | |

**Figure 7–6** General systems capabilities

| Ability to maintain the confidentiality of patient demographic, medical record, billing, and financial data belonging to each physician or group of physicians using the system, specifically: | | | | |
|---|---|---|---|---|
| Security-controlled access to patient and financial data by individual physician | | | | |
| Security-controlled access to patient and financial data by group/department | | | | |
| User flexibility in regard to which data/information is shared with other members of a group(s) | | | | |

**Figure 7–6** (continued)

- Description of the options available for upgrades to the proposed hardware configuration, as transaction volume increases and additional applications are installed, beyond those addressed in the RFP, for example, larger processor, more memory, additional processors

**Operating System and Utilities**

Obtain specific information in writing under each of the following categories:
- A description of any changes they have made to the standard operating system, communications software, or file access methods, indicating where these changes have been made and how these changes will affect future upgrades
- A description of the length and frequency of backup, restore, or reorganization procedures that would interfere with on-line availability, including the time of day these would normally occur

**Application Software**
- A comment on whether the source code is provided
- Description of the procedure they use when providing enhancements or additions to the applications
- A comment on whether the enhancements/additions to the product are included as part of the standard software application maintenance agreement
- An explanation of the procedure by which the source code can be obtained if the vendor no longer supports the system
- A description of any high-level report writer that may be available

## SPECIFIC APPLICATION CAPABILITIES

The vendor is asked to respond with regard to its capability to provide for the detailed requirements listed below. Please provide any supporting documentation that leads to more understanding of your system capabilities. Feel free to emphasize any additional capabilities that you feel distinguish you from other vendors offering similar systems. Attach an addendum, listing the costs of each proposed modification. Include the cost of the third-party software in Section VI.

| Capability Description | Currently available | Not available, but willing to provide | Not available not willing to provide | Comments |
|---|---|---|---|---|
| PATIENT REGISTRATION | | | | |
| Ability to create, update, and delete account and patient record and track the following: | | | | |
| Patient name | | | | |
| Patient billing address (4 lines) | | | | |
| Second patient address | | | | |
| Birth date (4 characters for year) | | | | |
| Sex | | | | |
| Relation to responsible party | | | | |
| Home phone number | | | | |
| Work phone number | | | | |
| Primary care doctor | | | | |
| Person responsible | | | | |
| Person responsible address (4 lines) | | | | |
| Nine digit ZIP code | | | | |
| Person responsible phone number | | | | |
| System assigned account number | | | | |
| Referral source | | | | |
| Occupation | | | | |
| Employer name | | | | |
| Employer address | | | | |
| Employer phone number | | | | |
| Marital status | | | | |
| Spouse's name | | | | |

**Figure 7–7** Specific application capabilities

## HARDWARE AND SYSTEM SOFTWARE CAPABILITIES

INTRODUCTION

This section addresses issues related to the hardware and software in the proposed system. The vendor is asked to provide information on the issues/questions identified, for the following areas of the vendor's proposed system:

    System Architecture
    System Performance
    System Migration

SYSTEM ARCHITECTURE

Based upon your understanding of the size, workload, and future requirements of General Hospital, describe the technical characteristics of the proposed system in each category:

    Hardware
    Operating System and Utilities
    Application Software
    Data Security
    Data Communication Security

The following questions should be specifically addressed for each category:

    Is the technology proprietary to your firm? If so, please elaborate.
    Is the technology the most currently available release?
    How long has the technology you use, been in use?
    As new technology becomes available, how quickly do you upgrade your system?

Hardware

    Provide the proposed hardware that you believe will be sufficient to meet the requirements described in this RFP. In addition, provide the potential maximum quantities recommended under the proposed configuration and the characteristics that apply to the various devices, for example, monochrome/color terminals, printer speed, disk drive capacity.

| | Proposed | Potential Max | Characteristics |
|---|---|---|---|
| cpu | _____ | _____ | _____ |
| network servers | _____ | _____ | _____ |
| video terminals | _____ | _____ | _____ |
| printer terminals | _____ | _____ | _____ |
| system printers | _____ | _____ | _____ |
| smart card readers | _____ | _____ | _____ |
| voice recognition | | | |
| comm. boards | _____ | _____ | _____ |
| entry devices | _____ | _____ | _____ |
| magnetic disk | | | |
| drives | _____ | _____ | _____ |
| controllers | _____ | _____ | _____ |
| optical disk | | | |
|    drives | _____ | _____ | _____ |
| controllers | _____ | _____ | _____ |
| tape drives | _____ | _____ | _____ |
| terminal controllers | _____ | _____ | _____ |
| local | _____ | _____ | _____ |
| remote | _____ | _____ | _____ |
| network boards | _____ | _____ | _____ |
| network routers | _____ | _____ | _____ |

**Figure 7–8** Hardware and system software capabilities

- Details of how the report writer is accessed, both in batch mode and on-line
- A copy of their standard software application maintenance agreement
- A summary of their yearly increases in maintenance fees over the past five years

### Data Security

- A description of the method that restricts access to files or database record segments—by application program, by individual, or by user class
- A comment on whether files can be accessed simultaneously in both batch mode and on-line
- A description of the procedures for expanding files or the database, and how often this is usually necessary

### Data Communication Security

- A description of the various levels of security provided for application terminals—by application, by function within the application, and by employment classification
- A comment on whether there is an automatic log-off feature, and if so, a description of how it works

## System Performance

Always include a system performance clause in the RFP. This puts you on record regarding your expectations for performance from the system. Vendors typically balk at responding to this, so do not be surprised if they are hesitant or refuse to respond. If they refuse to provide a performance guarantee, at least you have a basis for discussion, specifically of what you can reasonably expect from the system and the types of remedies that would be available if your expectations are not met. Better to have this discussion now than to wait until a problem arises.

A typical performance clause would read as follows:

The system must have a low incidence of failure and a short mean recovery time, at both local and remote locations. The vendor will be held solely responsible for the reliable operation of the system and all of its components. The expected minimum levels of performance are as follows:

- Unscheduled downtime for the entire system must not exceed 1% of the total time in any three-month period.
- Unscheduled downtime for any terminal workstation must not exceed 1% of total time.
- System recovery must not require more than two hours for any one failure.
- Average response time must not exceed two seconds, 95% of the time, between the hours of 7:00 A.M. and 6:00 P.M. on any given day. In any case, response time must never exceed five seconds.

Please specify under what conditions you would guarantee the above minimum level of system performance.

### System Migration

If you will be replacing an old system, ask the vendor to describe the typical scenario that would be followed in migrating from the existing software application to the new one. If there is not a current system, ask for a description of the implementation process.

## SOLICITATION OF VENDORS

Once the RFP is complete to the satisfaction of the system selection committee and information management steering committee, forward a copy to each vendor. Include a transmittal letter that outlines any of the ground rules that were not included in the RFP document or that need to be repeated for emphasis. Things to include are the numbers of copies to be submitted, the deadline for submission of the responses, and the voice and fax numbers of the contact person. It is good practice, though not always effective, to warn the vendors against contacting anyone else within the organization concerning this RFP. Some organizations go as far as to threaten automatic disqualification if this rule is violated. It is to your advantage to keep the process as equitable as possible, for as long as possible. Limiting the vendors' access reduces possible unfair advantage resulting from contacts cultivated outside the RFP process.

It is best to keep the number of vendors reasonably small. If the initial research into potential vendors, either through an RFI or other means, was thorough, you should have a good idea of the four or five most qualified vendors. Avoid opening the process to too many vendors. This is one instance where "the more the merrier" definitely does not apply.

## EVALUATING RESPONSES

Up to this point, every effort has been made to keep the selection process objective. Too often objectivity breaks down during the evaluation. This does not have to happen. In fact, it should never be allowed to happen. A lot of work has gone into the selection process so far, and it could all be wasted if objectivity becomes a casualty.

## Applying Weights

Prior to scoring the RFP responses, develop a worksheet. With the help of the information management steering committee, assign weights to the major applications in the RFP, reflecting their relative importance to one another and to the whole. The weights should be expressed in terms of a decimal fraction of 1. For example, if there were four major applications each weighted equally, each would have a weight of .25 ($4 \times .25 = 1$). The higher the weight, the greater the impact on the total score. The following are some things to be considered when assigning weights to applications:

- The application may represent one of the main reasons the system is being sought in the first place (heavily weighted)
- The application may be key to providing for the needs of future programs and services (heavily weighted)
- The application may be a new one to the vendors and, therefore, not yet well developed (lightly weighted)
- The application may be well established, such as *Patient Registration,* and therefore well developed by all vendors, providing little opportunity for differentiation (lightly weighted)

These weights will be used to determine a weighted score for each application area. The purpose of weighting the results is to ensure that a product that is very strong in an area of lesser importance, but weak in an area of great importance, is not given precedence.

## Scoring System Capabilities

Next, score the system capability requirements section of the RFP. This is the section in the "yes, no, maybe so" format. The vendor was asked to mark an "X" in whichever box applied. Give all the "yes" answers a score of 2, all the "maybe" answers a score of 1, and all the "no" answers a score of 0. Add the scores for each major section. These sections correspond to the applications, which have previously been assigned weights on the worksheets. For example, *Patient Registration* would have a score, *Scheduling* would have a score, *Order Entry* would have a score, and so on. Enter the actual scores in the worksheet. Divide the raw score for each application by the highest possible score for that application, then multiply the quotient by the weight assigned to that specific application (actual score ÷ highest possible score × weight). Total the weighted scores.

## Determining Overall Fitness

Review the answers to the questions in the RFP regarding hardware and software. Using a worksheet that reflects each question, indicate whether the response is "acceptable" or "not acceptable." There is no "right" answer to most of these questions. But a system, for example, that is designed to operate only in a mainframe environment would be unacceptable to an organization that was strictly client-server based. Much of what is contained in this portion of the RFP is important in assessing whether the vendor would fit well with the way you operate. Answers that appear to be unacceptable should be clarified with the vendor to eliminate any possible misunderstanding. If the vendor becomes the vendor of choice, you would want to resolve any outstanding "unacceptable" responses during contract negotiations.

## Comparing Configurations

Using a worksheet, summarize the proposed hardware and software configurations. Vendor responses to the same RFP often differ dramatically when it comes to their perception of what is needed for hardware and operating system software. Often, in an attempt to lower the perceived price of the system, vendors will understate the hardware requirements, anticipating that if selected, they would be reimbursed for upgrades based on "new information." Remember that the reason for the RFP in the first place is to avoid as much "new information" as possible after the purchase.

If the RFP was constructed with full detail on the expected volumes and workload, both current and future, the vendor should be able to size the proposed system accordingly. Proper sizing of the system is a burden that the vendor must be willing to accept. The vendors are the only ones in a position to judge how their product will fit into your stated environment. Different systems may not require the same amount of disk space because of different record sizes, file structures, and storage techniques, but two different systems should normally require the same number of terminal devices based on the number of users indicated in the RFP. Discrepancies in terminal devices are easy to spot and correct. Discrepancies in processor speed, memory, and disk space are not as easy to identify. For a fair comparison, however, these discrepancies must be eliminated. Obtain new quotes if necessary, and add them to the worksheet. Differences may be legitimate, but the vendor needs to provide assurance by agreeing to a specified performance warranty.

## Performance Warranties

Vendors all have legitimate concerns with performance warranties. In fact, be a little bit leery of a vendor that agrees to a performance warranty without hesitation. It is necessary to discuss the exact framework within which the warranty will be applied. Vendor concerns usually revolve around the operating environment. If there are other applications already running on the same platform as the one the vendor's products will use, the vendor cannot be expected to be accountable for performance problems that may be caused by a prior application. If the system is used much more intensely than the vendor anticipates, the response times could suffer. The number of users may be accurate, for example, but no one would anticipate that one hundred percent of those users would be using the same application at the same time. That would represent an inordinate level of intensity on one application. Figure 7–9, sample performance warranty contract wording, contains a warranty clause that was negotiated considering these concerns.

Summarize the system costs quoted in the RFP on another worksheet. Include all adjustments resulting from changes to the hardware or software configuration, or the vendor's services.

VENDOR warrants that the System sold hereunder will operate in accordance with the specifications and performance guarantees contained in the VENDOR response to Customer's RFP, included by reference as Attachment E, the VENDOR software User Documentation (Release _____ and above) included by reference as Attachment F, and the System Performance Schedule included by reference as Attachment G.; and that the system configuration contains all necessary hardware, software of VENDOR or software or operating software of any third party to conform to the technical specifications and performance guarantees for a five (5) year period from the date of acceptance.

VENDOR warrants that the electronic transmission of Medicare and Medicaid claims for the states of Kansas and Missouri will operate in accordance with the specifications for the states of Kansas and Missouri or the designated intermediary, and furthermore that the implementation of said transmission capability will be completed and available for use coincident with activation of the corporate-site system.

In the event that the System sold hereunder fails to meet the warranties under this agreement at any time during the first year following the final payment called for in Attachment E, VENDOR, at its expense and at Client's option, shall remedy the deficiency within thirty (30) days, a reasonable, mutually agreed upon, time period, following notification of the deficiency by Client.

In the event that the equipment sold hereunder fails to meet the performance warranties under this agreement at any time during a period of three (3) years following the final payment called for in Attachment E, VENDOR shall provide Client at VENDOR's expense, at Client's option, additional or replacement equipment sufficient to remedy the performance deficiency. Upon demonstration to Client's satisfaction that the performance requirements are being met, Client shall pay to VENDOR the then current direct cost to VENDOR of the additional computer equipment, exclusive of VENDOR's markups and installation fees.

**Figure 7–9** Sample performance warranty contract wording

## Determining Relative Value

Find the relative value score by dividing the total system capabilities score by the total cost of the system. While this number should not be used as the deciding factor in system selection, it is often instructive. Sometimes very similar capabilities can be purchased at very dissimilar prices. The relative value score highlights this and should prompt further investigation.

## "AND THE FINALISTS ARE"

Once all of the information provided in the RFPs is scored, clarified, adjusted, and documented on worksheets, identifying those systems and vendors worthy of further investigation is easy. From a field of five candidates, it is usually possible to identify the two or three you would like to invite for on-site product demonstrations.

Whatever the number, do not include any vendor beyond the point in the process where that vendor is no longer a viable candidate. It is a waste of everyone's time. It can become very expensive for vendors to participate in this process. Although they consider it as a normal cost of doing business, it is not ethical to have them continue when there is no hope of them winning the contract. They could be using those resources to pursue other future business. Remember, particularly during contract negotiations, the client-vendor relationship is symbiotic. It is in the client's interest for these system vendors to prosper, even those vendors that you do not choose.

## ON-SITE PRODUCT DEMONSTRATIONS

You will want to actually see the product. Before the advent of on-line systems, this was straightforward. Product review consisted of looking at the forms used for data entry and the reports generated by the system. This could be accomplished without the vendor's presence on site. Today, it is a little more complicated and a lot more expensive.

You will want the vendor to demonstrate the on-line capabilities of the system at a location that is convenient for many of your staff to attend. This usually means a large meeting room at a central location. If you belong to a multihospital organization, it is reasonable to request demonstrations at more than one site.

In setting up the demonstration, scale the audience and agenda to the equipment being used by the vendor. Many demonstrations are done on personal computers with fifteen-inch screens. No more than four or five people can comfortably view the screens at one time, so several sessions would need to be scheduled. If the image is projected onto a larger screen, a much larger audience can be accommodated, but audience participation is more limited.

In any event, control the demonstration. If you do not, the vendor will. This is a situation where your goals and the goals of the vendor will be different. It is all right to let the vendor get its points across, as long as you accomplish your goals as well.

Your demonstration goals should be:

- To get a good appreciation of the overall look and feel of the product
- To verify that the features that are of highest priority work the way you would expect them to work
- To discover weaknesses that are not apparent through the RFI and RFP responses
- To familiarize a wider audience with the system than that which has been involved up to this point
- To get a look at how the vendor performs

• To compare and contrast the software applications being demonstrated
• To move closer to final selection

The vendor's goals are:

• To differentiate themselves from the competition
• To build support from a wider audience for the system, than has been involved up to this point
• To emphasize the strengths of the system
• To emphasize the vendor's strengths
• To create a favorable impression of themselves and the product
• To move one step closer to a sale

Up to this point, the system evaluation has purposely been kept as objective as possible. Moreover, as far as possible, it is to the buyer's advantage to remain objective. Even now, there is no place for emotion.

Here is a story, whether true or not, that is unfortunately all too believable. Several years ago, a large medical center was in the market for a HIS. They were invited by a company to visit their offices in New York for a demonstration of the system. The first night in town, they were treated to a lavish dinner and drinks at a very expensive nightclub. The following morning, suffering from the effects of a late night and too much to drink, the visitors arrived late at the company offices. There was just enough time for a slide presentation on the company before lunch. Lunch was a banquet, lasting well into the afternoon. At its end, it was decided that there would be just enough time for everyone to go back to the hotel, make some calls home, take a short nap, freshen up, and get ready for dinner and a Broadway show.

The following day, the visitors had a 1 P.M. flight home. Morning meetings started at 9 A.M. They were introduced to the vendor staff who would be responsible for the account—an attractive and charming group. This was followed by a slide presentation of the future product development plans (it is amazing what you can do with slides), followed by a half-hour demonstration of the system itself, and a dash to the airport for the flight home.

Over the course of a two-day visit, they had a half-hour demonstration! Even more incredible, they bought the system—a five million dollar investment. Not so incredible, the implementation was a disaster. Most of the system they bought existed only on the overhead slides. The reasons they bought the system primarily had to do with good food and drink, first-class Broadway entertainment, and charming companionship.

This, to be sure, is an extreme example, but less obvious examples are quite common. It is all too easy and all too human to make emotional judgments based on how we feel toward the vendor representatives, the screen colors, the condition of the demonstration equipment, and the slide show presentation. Vendors know this and do their best to take advantage of it.

So, how do we help everyone focus on the merits of the system and the important attributes of the vendor? We enforce structure, just as we have in all previous steps of the selection process. No, it is not sexy. Yes, it is work. But it is worth it. The following section will tell you how to do it.

## ORGANIZING PRODUCT DEMONSTRATIONS

Control all aspects of the demonstration environment.

- Consult with the vendors to determine the appropriate time frame needed to fully demonstrate their systems. Provide as much time as they need within reason, and give each vendor the opportunity for equal time.
- To the extent possible, provide each vendor with the equipment they need to do a complete demonstration. You want to avoid having a vendor justify a second demonstration because of an avoidable problem.
- Schedule the demonstrations chronologically close together to minimize memory loss between demonstrations.

The selection committee should meet before each demonstration to review the RFP responses and agree upon important items that must be covered. Educate the audience beforehand, so they get the most out of each demonstration. Normally vendors will concentrate their demonstrations on routine activities that show their systems in the best light. Ask yourselves what benefits you hope to derive from the system and create written case scenarios for the vendor to follow. Scenarios should reflect problems you currently have that you hope to solve with the new software application.

Provide each attendee with an evaluation sheet for completion following each demonstration. Quantify the results on a scale of 1 to 10 (1 being worst, 10 being best) under the following categories:

- Overall look and feel of the software application
- Vendor's effectiveness in following case scenarios
- Satisfaction with the vendor's responses to questions and concerns
- Perceived appropriateness of the software application to the organization's needs
- Perceived ability of the vendor to meet the organization's needs

Once demonstrations are complete, the results have been quantified, and all follow-up questions have been answered, the system selection committee should meet to discuss the outcome and to plan site visits.

# SITE VISITS

Site visits may or may not be necessary. At this point, if you think you can reach a decision without going through this process, go for it. Site visits are difficult to coordinate around work schedules and can be expensive, depending on the number of people involved and the distances traveled.

If site visits are made, again structure the visits to get the most out of them. Everyone on the visit should take along a checklist of things to be covered. Some people like to have the vendor organize the visits, but leave the vendor behind for the actual visit. The hosts will be more open without the vendor present.

Our experience is that site visits, no matter how well organized, are of limited value. The operational environment in which these visits are made does not lend itself to critical evaluation. Normally space is limited, and a group of people hovering over a workstation rarely discovers anything meaningful. Host organizations are handpicked by the vendors and often feel it is an honor to be chosen. Therefore, they do not want to offend the vendor, and they treat the group like "company," putting on the best face possible. Even if they secretly feel they made a bad selection, they are more likely to admit this fact privately over the telephone than in person during a site visit.

# VENDOR REFERENCES

With or without site visits, always do a thorough job of calling references. If there is still concern over any aspect of the system or vendor, ask the references. Make an effort to contact references other than those provided by the vendor. These calls often produce the most candid responses.

# CHAPTER

# Contract Negotiations

*In life, you don't get what you deserve, you get what you negotiate.*
—P. Engel, *Negotiating.*

## REQUEST FOR PROPOSAL (RFP) AUDIT

The RFP audit is one of the most effective and rewarding exercises you can do. Properly conducted, the RFP audit provides value during both contract negotiations and product implementation.

Once the software application finalist has been selected, arrange to meet with the vendor to review, face-to-face, the vendor's specific responses to the RFP. The agenda of this meeting is to carefully review the RFP responses in order to ensure that the vendor interpreted the items in the RFP the way you intended, and to discover and remove any mistakes or misrepresentations.

It should not be surprising that there will be misrepresentations. Keep in mind that the vendor is responding to the RFP in a competitive situation. At the time of the RFP, the vendor's goal is to "stay in the game." To do so, the vendor will interpret the RFP items to its best advantage. Rightfully so, since the competition will do the same.

You do not want to be surprised by misrepresentations or misinterpretations later. Identify them now, so that remedial measures can be discussed during contract negotiations if necessary. Believe me, you will be well rewarded for the day or two spent on this exercise. We have been involved in many RFP audits, and every one of them has produced significant issues that later became items for discussion during contract negotiations. The vendor realizes that the sale is not closed yet, and is much more flexible about resolving these issues now than it will be after the sale.

This one exercise is best conducted on the vendor's turf. In addition to the sales staff that you have dealt with almost exclusively up to this point, you want the vendor's product implementation and support people involved as well. The product people are intimately familiar with the detailed design and functional characteristics of the product. They are held accountable for the promises made by the salespeople and, therefore, view the RFP responses from a much more pragmatic perspective. They are often able to respond to the feasibility of change requests on the spot. If they cannot make promises, at least they can gather all the information they need from you in order to research a request, without you having to go through an intermediary.

Keep in mind that after the contract is signed, the salespeople will disappear. The RFP audit is a good opportunity for you and the product people to get to know one another.

Make it clear that the RFP will be included as an attachment to the final contract. Therefore, the vendor will be held responsible for all representations contained in the RFP response. If you recall, this was made a condition of bidding in the sample RFP discussed earlier. When put in these terms, the vendor usually takes this exercise very seriously. This is the final opportunity for you and the vendor to fine-tune the response, to clearly represent what is needed and what will be delivered.

Review the RFP item by item, line by line. This can be long and tedious, but it is very important. Keep focused, and keep a master copy on which all changes are made, and have the vendor initial each change.

Upon completion of this exercise, you and the vendor will have a much clearer understanding of each other and the tasks that lie ahead. Items that materially deviate from the original RFP responses may become issues during contract negotiations. Keep track of these items for future discussions.

## NEGOTIATING THE CONTRACT

Negotiation is a skill we practice in our everyday lives. We ask family members what they want for dinner and may get several answers. The method of deciding what will be served is negotiation. In every negotiation, it is best to end up with a "win-win" solution. "Win-win" is beneficial to all parties. Everyone walks away feeling positive.

Success depends on all parties working toward the same goal. In negotiating, discussions should begin with "if, then" statements. For example, "If we can have meat loaf tonight, then I will be glad to make spaghetti tomorrow night."

We negotiate all the time. The same techniques can be used to negotiate the contract for a multimillion dollar Health Information System (HIS) for your health care organization. The most common misconception about contract negotiations is that because the contract becomes a legal document, you need a lawyer to do it. This could not be further from the truth. The contract is first a business document, containing business issues framed in a legal context. The business is primary; the legalities are secondary. Therefore, the people who understand the business and technical issues should carry out contract negotiations. Once those issues are settled to the satisfaction of all parties, the contract should then be sent to the lawyer to ensure the proper legal framework is in place as well.

Business issues likely to be addressed include:

• The hardware and software being acquired
• Software modifications
• Implementation and training responsibilities
• The implementation schedule
• Purchase price and payment schedule
• System performance warranties
• Product and service warranties
• Remedies in case of nonperformance by either party
• Remedies in the event the system performance warranties are not met

Legal issues will likely include:

• The state under whose law the contract terms will be governed (always make it your state, *not* the vendor's)
• The framework within which disputes will be resolved, either through the courts or through arbitration
• "Wordsmithing" into legal jargon comfortable to the legal establishment

## Selecting Your Team

Be very selective about your team. Make sure that the team members are prepared to go into the negotiations with confidence and knowledge. Include technical, business, and financial representatives who can speak with authority for your organization. These members should have a clear understanding of what it is your institution needs from this product. They should be schooled in the functions and features presented in the product demonstrations. They should be excited about the purchase of the product, but cautious about the process. They will probably be individuals who have been involved in the selection from the beginning.

## Preparing Your Team

Meet as a team before the negotiations. Discuss and agree upon your overall negotiating plan.

- Understand what is possible with the product.
- Agree on which functions and features are important to the organization.
- Prioritize: make a list of all the items you must have, followed by those you would like to have in order of decreasing importance.
- Agree on second choices. For each item you have decided you must have and would like to have, create a "fall back" level of acceptance.
- Agree on low priority needs. Make a list of "painless concessions"—items that you do not really care about and that would not be painful to give up.
- Agree on nonnegotiable items. Determine these items and understand that, once identified, they can have the effect of forcing both parties to be more flexible on other issues that are negotiable.

Your expressed concerns regarding the vendor's nonnegotiable items can serve as bargaining chits, even if you secretly do not care about these items. Use this to your advantage; the vendor will do the same to you. Nonnegotiable items can be showstoppers if a compromise cannot be reached.

## Negotiating Techniques

The following are negotiating techniques often used by negotiators. Some of them require practice to be done effectively. Being perceived as competent, businesslike, and sincere is of primary importance. Do not do anything that would jeopardize that perception.

- Try to anticipate the vendor's point of view on the issues and agree in advance about what your position will be.
- Do not be afraid to ask for things that may seem outrageous. The more times the vendor says "no," the greater the pressure on the vendor to appear to be negotiating in good faith, and the greater the likelihood that you will get a concession on something of real importance to you.

- Deal only with someone at a level that can legitimately assume decision making. Otherwise you will waste time going back and forth getting approvals for every concession you request.
- Develop team consensus. Do not allow dissension within the ranks, at least in view of the vendor. If a potential disagreement among your team members arises, ask for a recess and discuss it out of earshot.
- Do not allow winks, urgent scribbling, staring, frowns, embarrassed smiling, and so on among the members of the team at the table. A courteous businesslike attitude will be appreciated and reciprocated. Remember the saying, "You can catch more flies with honey than with vinegar."

You, acting as the team manager, should involve all members in playing different roles in the negotiation process. However, you are the one who makes the final decisions. You must feel comfortable with any negotiating techniques you decide to use. Common ones are listed in the following text, but do not use any of them if you do not think you can pull them off. You do not want to embarrass yourself by being perceived as trying to be too "cute." Remember, the vendor does this all the time and knows that you do not. It is better to come across as a sincere amateur than as a foolish one.

### Good Guy–Bad Guy

Role-play. Practice. You must have a partner who can believably act out one role. The bad guy role is more difficult to perform. Both partners should agree exactly on the mission of this role-play. Work out hand signals for concepts like:

- "Make note, try again later"
- "Push harder"
- "Softer"
- "Let me take over"

In dealing with the vendor, you may encounter a variety of posturing techniques. The following text describes some of the most common.

### Stonewalling

This is characterized by people who do not change their minds, reduce their demands, or provide flexibility. It is exactly the opposite of what negotiations are supposed to be—even-handed, fair-minded, and give-and-take. Break through the stone wall by:

- Verifying that your offer is reasonable
- Setting limits on negotiations and breaking them off if necessary

- Asking the vendor to justify any unwillingness or to explain why they are acting this way

## *Bluffing*

A bluff is a false statement, usually an exaggeration, about what may occur if you do not do something. Some negotiators bluff intensely; if you suspect this, call them on it. These are false statements, and one wonders about dealing with a person who is intentionally lying during negotiation of a business relationship.

Sometimes the bluff is for only a short time. For example, "Call me by tomorrow morning or I will get on the plane." You need to decide whether this is real, and what it would mean to you if the person got on the plane.

If you bluff, the other side can refuse to concede and call your bluff, catching you in a lie. If you get caught, be clear about your next option.

## *Bad Temper*

Bad temper is a characterization of a negotiator who is in a bad mood, ill-tempered, or may be just plain nasty. Here are two approaches to handle this:

- Fight fire with fire. It is difficult for anyone to be mean and bad-tempered for an extended period of time, and it is probably not effective for two people to fight it out at a negotiating table. Ask that another time to be set for negotiations, or ask for a different negotiator.
- Assume a caretaker role. You can offer sympathy and show concern to this person, since everyone has bad days, but do not let this intimidate you or make you stray from the agenda.

## *Intimidation*

This occurs when negotiators threaten to bring in the big guns in order to get what they want. Some suggestions for this:

- Do not show any response to threats.
- Cancel negotiations. Be careful; you may have to cancel, but then that may be okay if things have gotten this bad.
- With a take-it-or-leave-it attitude, that is, "this is our best offer," you can respond by:
  — Ignoring it and acting as if you never heard the statement—continuing to negotiate
  — Sending back your own statement just like it—appearing angry and offended and calling them on their offer

— Demanding a good faith concession
— Submitting to their demands

### *Back Pedaling*

This occurs when one side feels it has given up too much or promised something it cannot produce and tries to find a way to explain why things have changed. You may hear excuses such as:

• My needs have changed.
• My situation has changed.

## Negotiating Tips

Give your team training in communication; keep the group tight. Remind the team members of the skills needed for negotiation, which can include:

**Debate.** Listen carefully to what the opponent is saying. Find strength and weaknesses in their arguments and their facts. Determine what issues and arguments are most important to your position. Prioritize these points. Plan defense and offense surrounding these points.

**Straw Man.** Argue another less important issue to focus attention away from the main issue. If you are arguing, this gives you time to regroup. If the opponent is arguing, however, this wastes your time and you need to bring them back to the real issue.

**Change the Subject.** For example, "That reminds me of. . . ." This uses up valuable time, forcing the opponents to extend their schedule, giving you more time for investigation or planning strategies. If it is the vendor attempting to waste time, again, you must bring them back to the point at hand.

**Questioning.** By posing a series of questions, you can lead opponents to conclusions just by them answering correctly. This is very difficult, but if done well, it is very difficult to argue against.

Rehearse negotiation scenarios beforehand.

Determine whether you are negotiating from a strong or a weak position. You are in a position of strength if you have more options than the other party and cannot be forced into accepting the other side's terms. Evaluate your opponent's "strengths" by determining:

• How easy it is for them to get what they want from others
• Whether you will survive without the products or services received from them

A party negotiating from a weak position has fewer options and possibly can be forced into accepting the other side's terms. Evaluate what you have to lose and the timing of the negotiations. Two tactics that can be used:

- Refuse to reach agreement, and your opponent must begin over again. You may become known as a "difficult client."
- Decline to meet the timetable for giving the other side what they want. Stalling can be effective, but be clear about what it is you are trying to gain.

Four ways to strengthen a weak position:

1. Determine how much your opponent needs you. Research this beforehand.
2. Explore ways to improve your position by temporarily modifying your product or service, reducing the price, and so on.
3. Imply there are others who are interested in you and your business.
4. Treat *every* concession you must make like it is a huge concession.

Review good active listening skills with your team: evaluate what you have heard, weigh the information, decide how to use it, and then react. More than one-third of our time is spent listening. Active listening helps the group stay focused and centered on one issue (Patterson, 1996). Some suggestions to review with your group:

- Maintain good eye contact, smile, nod, and behave as if you find the opponent's argument persuasive.
- Pay close attention to each speaker; resist distractions.
- Listen to the words carefully and the way they are being used; judge content, not delivery.
- Watch the opponent's body language. Evaluate for:
  — Posture: erect, upper body leaning forward indicates readiness, action, and alertness
  — Facial expression: animation in facial expression and good eye contact shows interest
  — Tone of voice: voice is audio to the face, conveying emotion, honesty, and vulnerability in depth
  — Position: crossed arms and legs indicate withdrawal and defensiveness. Open posture shows a more respectful attitude

Analyze the thinking that lies beneath your opponent's position on each point. Listen between the lines. Do not think about your reaction just yet; do not argue or judge until you comprehend. If you find your attention slipping, call a break and refresh yourself. Do not be overpowered by marathon sessions.

Negotiate only one point at a time. Ask three questions about each point:

- What are you looking for here?
- How can we come to terms on this point?
- What is your bottom line on this item?

Ask these questions several times during the negotiations, and listen for changes in answers as the talks continue.

Take careful notes of what is said and refer to them often. Write your negotiable targets on 3" × 5" cards, and keep the cards with you at the table. Refer to them frequently. Make your notes on them. Be creative in taking notes—listen for central themes, not just facts. Focus time and energy on negotiable targets, and as each is completed, write down the conclusion and move on to the next point. Check back through cards before signing the contract to review concessions.

When you find an item the opponent does not want to negotiate:

- Focus time and energy on this issue and find out why it is not negotiable.
- Make this issue central to all negotiations.
- Keep coming back to other party's refusal to negotiate this issue, and use it as evidence that you are being asked to give up more than the other party because of this refusal.

Do not be intimidated by expensive clothing and briefcases. Picture these people as just another person—getting paid to do a job, just as you are.

Clear communication is necessary. Veteran negotiators may "intentionally" misunderstand you, mislead you, and try to gain advantage, create confusion, or win concessions. Be careful to move from point to point, carefully making notes as you go for review later. Practice conversations with your team. Be careful and very clear about:

- What point you are presently discussing—stick with that item until it is finished, or make note of it and table it until later
- Pointing out each offer you make to the other side
- What objections your side has given to the offer, either in its entirety or item by item
- What changes will facilitate this agreement
- When you move from one discussion point to another
- The agenda—keep goals in front of you. Make notes as needed concerning specific items. Refer to *your* goals when new topics come up and the conversation

changes. If a new topic is more directly related to a major goal of yours, pursue it. If not, then it is probably a distraction and you need to refer the conversation back to your major point being discussed

Beware of responses like:

- "That's all well and good, but first we really need to concentrate on . . ."
- "I can agree to that matter, provided you say yes right now to my suggestions regarding . . ."
- "That issue will probably take care of itself, once we agree on . . ."

Practice a judicious pause. Breathe before you speak. Listen carefully and actively. If you suspect there is misunderstanding on a point, stop and return to that point and clarify it again. If necessary, write points of agreement out and ask for your opponent's initials.

Wait for the other party to finish. There is great value in letting the other party talk and talk, until they wind down. Many times, you hear different things the second or third time through that were not there for the first rendition. Listen for them. Make notes and confront them as necessary.

Do not ask yes or no questions. For example, "Can you reduce the price by $10?" Instead say, "What is your position on discounting the price to us?" Be persistent; keep coming back to the question that will get the answers you want and need. If you are told, "Gee, I don't know, I'll have to get back to you," make note of that and ask again after the break.

Make your arguments persuasive. Insert information. Back up your facts with reference books, quotations, photographs, articles, and so on. You will gain credibility if you bring in experts for key arguments.

Downplay your weaknesses. Do not, however, ignore them or deny them. If you do, they will only get bigger.

## Approaching the Negotiating Table

Control the conference space. If you can, set up the meetings in very comfortable and pleasant surroundings. Depending on the table configuration, you want the position of power. If it is a long table, sit at one end and seat your team members on either side of you. If it is a round table, sit opposite the door, in the middle of the table, again, with your team members on either side of you. Make sure the lighting is moderate, not too bright, as in interrogation, but not too dark, increasing the chances of players dozing off.

Meals may be served. Roll out the red carpet. Ask if there are dietary restrictions for any of the vendor's team members. Make sure there is coffee and tea in the morning, water, and sodas in the afternoon. Keep meals light and healthy, decreasing the amount of lag that occurs after a heavy meal. We do not recommend alcohol when you want your performance at its peak.

When scheduling negotiations, it is to your advantage to have the meeting at your site. Think of it as your home court; it has all the support that comes with that advantage. Several factors to keep in mind when making this decision:

- **Adequate Sleep.** You and your team are sleeping at your homes in your own beds. There are no time changes or jet lag to deal with.
- **Experts/User Resources.** Your experts/users can be readily available and called in, if changes to the contract are necessary.
- **Pace.** Because it is your home court, you are in control and can proceed at a pace that is comfortable for you and your team members.
- **Bargaining Incentive.** Because the vendor has traveled to your site and is spending expense dollars to support its team, the team members may be more willing to negotiate the contract within a short time frame in order to meet airline schedules, other contract meetings, and so on.

If you decide that you want to negotiate your contract at the vendor's offices, be aware of the same considerations and be a smart traveler:

- Take early flights. Make sure that you and your team get enough rest. Avoid late nights.
- Prepare: before the negotiation begins, meet with your team and go over strategy.
- Stay in close contact with your health care organization, keeping them apprised of progress and any changes that may occur. Telephone calls are cheap when we are talking about millions of dollars.
- Be prepared to take as much time as needed to get the best deal. Keep focused on the negotiations.

Be aware of deadlines. Nothing is ever decided early on in negotiations. There is power in using deadlines. Be careful not to allow the other side to set them or to let them intimidate you. Make deadlines benefit you:

- Set the negotiation deadline yourself.
- Let your opponent know you are not available after this deadline.
- Find a deadline that naturally exists, such as a holiday, fixed deadline, trade show, convention, and so on.

• Ask for a deadline from your opponent. This is used effectively if you are having a problem with their service: "How long do you think I should tolerate this poor service you are giving me?"

Keep your expectations of the negotiation reasonable. Remember the best solution to a negotiation is a win-win. Think through these five areas before signing a contract:

• **Money.** Everyone or everything should have a cost in direct proportion to the value of the contribution made.
• **Power.** Determine who has influence over final product, design, and decision.
• **Options.** Be reasonable. Think of what is "usual and normal" in most cases. Do not get caught in fixed solutions.
• **Rights and Responsibilities.** Make sure those who are expected to do something have the means and authority to do it.
• **Ownership.** There will be ownership. Who will own what?

## Offer and Acceptance

In a system negotiation, there are many items, such as price, deliverables, schedules, warranties, and remedies, to be negotiated. As you negotiate each item, and as you are nearing the end of the negotiation, think about your offer. If you can help it, do not be the first to make a final offer. Once you have made the final offer, the other side has twice as much information as you do. They now know your bottom line, as your offer usually gives them an idea of what your bottom line is. Here are some suggestions:

• Make a strategic offer. You may lowball your offer, and the opponent may respond with a counteroffer. When you offer first, their counteroffer may still not reveal their bottom line.
• Counteroffers put you on the defensive. The vendor's representatives keep all their information close to the vest and simply work with *your* original offer.
• If you must offer first, offer to concede something small.

Here are three ways to untangle who offers when:

1. Ask for an offer straight out. If they offer at this point, you win.
2. Delay, delay, and delay. Simply do not make offers yourself.
3. Play hardball:
   • Suggest that "we do not have all the details."
   • "There are so many intangibles here. . . ."
   • "We are here to see what arrangement you are offering us."

Here are some tips on how and when to offer concessions:

• Offer your concessions in reverse priority order, with the least important one first.
• Make every concession contingent on getting something else in return.
• Behave as though every concession is a loss of something vital from your side.

## The Contract

Once the details seemingly have been hammered out, review the contract to determine how well your organization is protected by this agreement. Ask these questions:

• What if they do not live up to this agreement?
• What is the worst possible scenario?
• How likely are they to:
    — fail to deliver the products or services in an acceptable form?
    — fail to perform on schedule?
    — fail to meet performance warranties?

With these questions answered, discuss how well you are protected in your agreement. What are your options? What recourse does it give you? Does it compensate for lost time or business?

If you are negotiating by phone:

• Take notes. Write down agenda items, and work from them.
• Ask for help. Use a speaker phone.
• Get interrupted, on purpose if necessary, so you can take a break.
• Hang up—end the conversation if you need to, and schedule another call.

In the final contract, remember to include references and attachments for the following:

• Itemization of hardware and software being purchased with corresponding prices
• Implementation schedule
• A payment schedule tied to milestones in the implementation schedule
• The audited and signed vendor response to the RFP
• Written specifications for product modifications and interfaces

In the end, all of the negotiating ploys and strategies in the world will do you no good if you end up with an agreement that either party is unhappy with. Remember, you are striving for a "win-win" result. You and your organization want to obtain good value for your investment. The vendor wants a good client. These are both achievable goals.

Once the contract is signed, the real work begins. The implementation effort is a partnership between you and the vendor. You begin building that partnership during contract negotiations.

# REFERENCES

Engel, P. (1996). *Negotiating.* Los Angeles: McGraw-Hill.

Patterson, J. G. (1996). *How to become a better negotiator.* New York: AMACOM.

# CHAPTER

# Implementation

It is to your benefit to obtain an implementation plan for attachment to the contract. Payments to the vendor under the contract can then be tied to certain milestones in the plan. Money is a great motivator to ensure that the vendor lives up to its commitments. This will require planning sessions with the vendor before or during contract negotiations.

Another benefit of doing this early is that you gain exposure to the vendor's implementation personnel and their approach before you have a signed contract. There was one instance where the customer was so offended by the vendor's heavy-handed approach to implementation that the customer decided against buying the software product. It was fortunate that this happened prior to signing the contract.

Vendors are usually reluctant to participate in implementation planning before they have a final agreement. If necessary, offer to break out the planning process into a separate engagement so the vendor can be assured of reimbursement for its efforts. Reduce the total value of the main contract by this amount. Be willing to give up this investment if negotiations do not work out.

# IMPLEMENTATION PLANNING

The first step in implementation planning is to identify the implementation team. The team should include a project leader, individuals familiar with the business and clinical operations that are the subject of the product being acquired, vendor product experts, and technical resources. Ideally, all of the team members should be identified in advance of planning, so they can all participate. By participating in the identification, discussion, and scheduling of tasks, each member gives an implicit commitment to the rest of the team that the member will complete tasks within the time frame agreed upon and set forth in the plan. If a plan is developed in the absence of the team members, they will not feel the same obligation.

# BENEFITS OF PROJECT PLANNING

Every project, regardless how small, should have a project plan. Just the fact that it has been defined as a project indicates that the activities involved are complex enough to warrant a plan.

The project plan helps us crystallize our thinking. It is natural to minimize the extent of the overall effort. Who can say that they have never underestimated the amount of work or time involved in getting a project done? More often than not, things take twice as long as we expect them to. By outlining, in detail, the tasks to be done and the estimated length of time involved, we are forced to view the project realistically.

A realistic plan is a great arbiter of expectations. In this role, it serves as a communication tool. In the beginning of a project, the plan can be used to convince others in the organization to be realistic in regard to time frames and the required resources. Throughout the project, the plan serves as an effective vehicle for status reporting. Not doing a plan does not change what is actually required; it only sets the participants up for future surprises and disappointments, or worse, failure.

A good project plan is effective in defending against that insidious enemy of all systems projects, "project creep." Project creep occurs when a project has not been well defined and controlled. New requirements are continuously being introduced. The project expands well beyond its original scope, and ultimately seems like it will never end. To make things worse, since the project was not well defined from the beginning, it is difficult to communicate to top management why the project is so over budget and behind schedule. An automated project-scheduling program is an indispensable tool for this process. There are many good ones on the market, costing about three to five hundred dollars, for use on a personal computer.

As the project leader, develop a high-level outline of the plan first, then meet with your project team to fill in the details. The team members are usually the experts. If the plan is for implementation of a vendor-supplied system, use the vendor's generic plan as a starting point, but do not ever use a vendor plan as the final version. I have yet to see a vendor-supplied plan that comprehensively includes both the vendor installation tasks and the customer implementation tasks.

Vendor plans include those activities that are universally required to *install* the software application or system. Installation includes tasks, such as configuring hardware, loading software, building files and tables, setting up interfaces, training users in the mechanics of the system, and file conversion. All of these are important tasks, to be sure, but they do not include those activities required to *implement* the system in your environment. Implementation activities include such things as developing procedures, redesigning work flow, developing forms, developing standards, and training the users to use the software within the context of the operating environment. The goal of a system implementation is to seamlessly integrate the software tool into the operating environment. Every environment is different; as a result, the vendor's universal plan needs to be tailored to fit.

## PLANNING GUIDELINES

Use the following nine guidelines in sequence when developing a plan. In fact, it is best to act on each guideline individually to the exclusion of the others, as you progress down the list. In that way, your judgment will be influenced only by considerations that are relevant to each step. For example, list all activities first before estimating the time required for each activity. If you do not do it this way, and the estimate is made at the same time each task is identified, you may unconsciously omit tasks as you begin to realize that the project is going to take longer than you had hoped. It would be easy to become mentally tired and discouraged.

1. Define the project boundaries.
2. Break projects into manageable pieces.
3. List activities.
4. Identify important milestones.
5. Estimate activity duration.
6. Assign dependencies between tasks.
7. List available resources.
8. Define expectations of all involved.
9. Never set target dates until all tasks have been estimated and assigned.

### Define Project Boundaries

Too often the boundaries of a project are fuzzy or not well defined. This is the biggest single contributor to "project creep." Even projects that implement vendor-provided software can become victims. The vendor knows when they are done, usually this time frame coincides with the final payment, but because this is an implementation, and not an installation, you may not be done.

From the beginning, identify an event that, on completion, will signal the end of the project, and stick to it. If additional tasks are identified during the course of the project, start a new project and call it phase 2. Phase 1 could be the original implementation project, phase 2 could be the enhancement project, and phase 3 could be the maintenance project. There is nothing more demoralizing than a project that seems to go on and on.

Sometimes identifying the beginning of a project is just as difficult as identifying the end. Identifying the beginning is important because this is the point at which you are lining up the resources and obtaining the authority to proceed.

Often system initiatives begin with a feasibility study. This study is conducted to determine whether there is a legitimate need; to investigate the options available to answer the need; and to estimate the money, material, and personnel resources that would be required to pursue each option. The feasibility study, in itself, is a project. Once approval is given to proceed on one of the options, pursuit of that option is an entirely separate project. Too often there is no differentiation between the feasibility study and the start of the main project. This can create confusion over roles, responsibilities, and authority for each project.

For each new project, ask the following questions:

• What do we intend to accomplish?
• Is this really more than one project?
• Under what conditions will we consider the project started?
• Under what conditions will we consider the project complete?
• Where will development/implementation end and maintenance begin?

## Break Projects into Manageable Pieces

Large projects can be very difficult to visualize when observed as a whole. In order to effectively estimate all the tasks involved, we need to visualize the problem. By breaking large projects into smaller pieces, we can visualize one piece at time and join the pieces to form the whole later. Look for natural boundaries. Almost every systems project, for example, has hardware, operating system software, application system software, and an implementation component. The project can be separated into smaller pieces at these boundaries.

An implementation project can be divided by functional grouping or by department, as in the examples for a laboratory system implementation in Figure 9–1. In Example 1, the implementation is defined in terms of the major systems activities to be carried out in each department. In Example 2, the same implementation is defined in terms of each

***Install Lab System*** could be broken down several ways:
  1. By site
  2. By major activity for the entire lab
  3. By department within the lab

**Example 1:**
  1. Chemistry
     Load software
     Define file structure
     Accumulate procedures
     Build procedure files
     Build ordering screens
  2. Hemo
     Load software
     Define file structure
     Accumulate procedures
     Build procedure files
     Build ordering screens

**Example 2:**
  1. Load software
     Chemistry
     Hemo
  2. Define file structure
     Chemistry
     Hemo
  3. Accumulate procedures
     Chemistry
     Hemo

**Figure 9–1** Break projects into manageable pieces

department and its corresponding systems activities. In the first example, the software would be implemented in one department at a time. In the second example, the software would be implemented across the entire laboratory at the same time.

## List Activities

As mentioned earlier, it is important to complete this activity to the exclusion of everything else. You do not want concerns about duration, scheduling, and personnel to cloud the picture. Ask your project team to list every possible activity they can think of that is related to the major tasks in the plan. Installing hardware, for example, is a major task that involves many different activities. Have the individuals who will be responsible for this task list everything that needs to be done to accomplish it. At this point, the list does not have to be in sequence. That exercise comes later. Encourage them to get as detailed as possible. The greater the detail, the easier it will be to make estimates in the next step.

When listing activities, it is easiest to move from the broadest scope into ever-increasing detail. For implementation plans of vendor-supplied software, the generic vendor plan is useful as a starting point for identifying detailed activities.

This is where the automated project-scheduling program becomes indispensable. Enter the program into the system. Start each activity with an action verb. Doing so helps crystallize the activity to its essence. For example, "Attach terminators to cables on 2-South nursing unit" describes the task unambiguously, and the task can be easily estimated, assigned, and verified when the time comes. On the other hand, "Terminator work on the 2-South nursing unit" is vague and open to different interpretations.

## Identify Important Milestones

Milestones serve as checkpoints by which to monitor progress along the way. Completion of the cabling activities on 2-South may be considered a milestone. If the work is completed on time or ahead of schedule, you will know that, at least for this part of the plan, you are on schedule. If the work is finished late, you will want to evaluate whether this is an anomaly and not likely to continue, or whether this is a pattern that needs to be corrected. Milestones are also useful references for status reporting.

Milestones should be significant events within the plan. Once all the activities have been identified, put them in chronological order. Identify blocks of activities that on either initiation or completion will represent a significant event. "Begin training" and "end training," for example, are both activities that represent significant events.

## Estimate Activity Duration

Once you have compiled an exhaustive list of activities, you are ready to make estimates of the length of time required for each activity. Automated scheduling programs allow you to express estimates in terms of hours, days, weeks, and months. We have found that for most projects in the health care setting, estimates that are made in day units are the easiest to track. Eight hours is considered one day, four hours is considered half a day, and so on. Keep in mind that an eight-hour day includes any downtime during the day for breaks and meetings, and that in many cases, project members have other duties outside this project. Also, remember to factor holidays and vacation time into the estimates.

Duration may be expressed in two ways, either in terms of actual time spent on an activity, or in terms of elapsed time required to accomplish the activity. Implementation plans should be estimated based on the actual time required for each activity. Elapsed time estimates are best for high-level planning, with no resource assignments. Be consistent with the unit of estimate, and the approach you decide upon, throughout the plan.

Project tracking occurs at the lowest level of detail, and that is the level at which the estimates should be made. The automated project scheduler will use the estimates at the lowest level and roll them up to the next level automatically.

## Assign Dependencies Between Tasks

To this point, the detailed tasks have been treated as if they are completely independent of one another. In practice, there are many interdependencies among the project tasks that need to be reflected in the plan.

Certain tasks need to be completed before other tasks can begin. For example, the hardware needs to be installed and operational, before the software can be loaded. This is referred to as a "finish-to-start" relationship. The finish of the first task triggers the beginning of the second.

Other tasks may need to start before a second task can start. The cabling needs to start, for example, before the terminals can begin to be connected. It is not necessary, however, to complete all the cabling before the terminal connections can begin. This is called a "start-before-start" relationship. In this case, we would probably delay the beginning of the terminal connections by a few days to give the cabling people an advance.

A variation of the start-before-start relationship is the "parallel" relationship. This occurs when both activities either need to be started and completed at the same time, or are completely independent of one another and, therefore, it does not matter if they are taking place at the same time.

Project scheduling software is not able to determine the true relationship between tasks on its own. Initially, tasks will be assumed to be either all in parallel to one another or in a finish-to-start relationship. The actual relationships need to be defined by you, using the tools provided within the scheduler. For each activity, ask these questions:

- What task must be completed before the next activity can start?
- What must start before this activity can start?
- Are there other activities that must/may be done in parallel to this activity?
- Is there a specific date upon which this activity must start or finish?

When assigning dependencies, remember to begin at the highest level and progress to the lowest levels of detail.

## List Available Resources

At this point, you are ready to assign responsibility for the tasks outlined in the plan. Resource assignment is one of the capabilities offered by scheduling packages; however, we do not recommend using it. Managing resources through one of these products is very complex and time-consuming. This function is intended for large, complex development projects that require an hourly accounting of time for billing or accounting purposes. Some of the functions are designed specifically for use by contractors working for the Department of Defense. For the types of projects done in most health care settings, it is much more effective to just make a notation on each of the tasks, with the initials of the responsible party, and track it manually.

When making assignments, be realistic about the availability of the resources being assigned. For each individual, take into consideration competing projects, other maintenance or support responsibilities, and vacations and holidays that could influence the percentage of time the individual can contribute to this project.

## Identify and Define Roles

Everyone involved in the project should clearly understand his role from the beginning. Misunderstandings and miscommunication can be avoided. Many roles are clarified when tasks are assigned; however, there are often individuals and groups involved in projects with no specifically assigned tasks. Most often, these resources are those being relied upon to provide approvals, oversight, and information, but sometimes they may be technical personnel who have no direct responsibility to the project but who will be relied upon in a consulting capacity. These might include:

- Administration
- Users
- Steering committees
- Coordinators or liaison representatives
- Database administrators, network administrators, computer operators, systems programmers

It is useful to identify as many of these people as possible and invite them to a meeting in which you explain the project and its scope, and define the roles everyone will be expected to play.

## Set Target Dates

There may be a generally accepted target date for completion of the project that was set before planning began. Often these dates are preset based on external events over which you have no control, such as the opening of a new clinic or the expiration of the maintenance agreement on the product being replaced. Even so, *never set target dates until all tasks have been estimated and assigned.* If you do so, you are inviting failure.

Artificial target dates can be deadly. The plan you develop should be viewed as a "reality check" on the feasibility of the preset date. If the planning has been done properly, with no regard for a preset target date, you will be rewarded with an end date to the plan that should be your actual target date for completion.

"Okay," you say, "that may be fine in a perfect world, but we do not live in one." That is true; often preset target dates cannot be overridden. But that does not have to be the end of the story. Once the plan is complete, you have a lot of information available to you that was not available before. Explore the following possibilities if the planned end date, as calculated by the scheduling software, is significantly further away than the preset date:

- *Is the preset date an arbitrary target that was set without a full appreciation of the work involved?*

  That is the first possibility you should explore. Often dates are tossed out because they sound good at the time, but there is no compelling reason why it *must* be that date. This, of course, is the circumstance that we all hope for, because it is easy to set new expectations based on the more realistic date produced by the plan. Unfortunately, it often does not turn out that way. The preset date may be there for a good reason and cannot be changed.

- *Can the plan be separated into phases, with phase 1 delivering the essential elements required to satisfy the target date, and subsequent phases completing the project as originally planned?*

  This approach is often a possibility because systems usually provide more capability than is minimally required. Using the project plan as a guide, you can often split out those tasks that will deliver the basic capability needed by the target date. This approach will extend the length of the overall project because it is less efficient. Tasks that are done in phase 1 may have to be repeated in subsequent phases.

- *Can additional resources be added to the plan to speed things up?*

  This is the least desirable of the options, for several reasons. Adding people increases the cost. In today's health care environment, people resources are usually scarce. There is a limit on how much time can be gained by adding more people. But there are time frames that can be shortened by adding staff. Hardware configuration and cabling can be staffed more heavily or contracted out. Table and file building responsibilities can broaden. Training can be scheduled in double or triple sessions.

The important thing to appreciate is that without a plan that is constructed originally without regard to a preset target date, you are taking a wild guess. At least with a plan, there is a basis for discussion and analysis of options. Usually, when the plan is presented in a well-thought-out fashion, reasonable heads will prevail and alternatives will be worked out. No one wants to be part of a suicide mission.

## ORGANIZING THE PROJECT

The project team, like teams for all information management projects, should fall under the direction of the information management steering committee. This committee should be composed of individuals with the authority to provide direction and commit resources to the project. The steering committee is the keeper of the information management plan and, therefore, understands the relationship of all information management projects.

### Information Management Steering Committee

This committee is formed to ensure that information management activities proceed in accordance with the strategic, operational, and financial goals of your organization. There should be representation from across the continuum of care. Include people from the following disciplines as permanent members:

• Administration
• Nursing
• Physicians
• Information technology department
• Health information management department
• Library services

The steering committee reports to the executive board. It establishes goals for productivity and quality improvement in an annual plan that are consistent with and supportive of the mission statement developed by the executive board. Members must have the authority to change operating priorities, reallocate resources, and reorganize teams and support teams on their own (Hradesky, 1998).

This main committee will have several work groups responsible for projects. Information management steering committees have a tendency to stop meeting after large implementations are complete. There seems to be so much focus on this main project that all the rest of the work is tabled and forgotten. Although this committee is a central focus during implementations, it has many other areas of responsibility that must be addressed as an ongoing and permanent committee. These are some of the ongoing responsibilities:

- Reviews the corporate strategic plan annually
- Reviews and updates the information management plan annually based on the corporate strategic plan, and as new projects are presented throughout the year
- Monitors the progress of the information management plan throughout the year
- Reviews, tests, and updates system disaster recovery plan annually
- Reviews, approves, and prioritizes information management projects
- Oversees the writing, review, and revision of all information management policies once every three years, or when necessary
- Oversees the writing, review, and revision of manual and automated forms for the organization to ensure consistency throughout the continuum of care
- Oversees security and confidentiality issues concerning the medical record or patient privacy
- Oversees medical record delinquency issues
- Monitors reporting to regulatory agencies
- Responsible for meeting and maintaining compliance with JCAHO information management standards
- Appoints project leaders and approves team members
- Provides guidance to project teams by:
  — Providing direction, resources, and support
  — Approving closure of each step
  — Developing plans to recognize and reward performance

Committees may be made up of as few as four or five people, or as many as twenty to twenty-five members in very large multisite organizations. The old adage "the more, the merrier" does not hold true here. Manageable numbers are needed. Committees are functional, given the "right" people, when there are eight to ten members. Again, the agenda should be rich in activities. This meeting should always start on time, and attendance sign-in sheets and meeting minutes should be recorded. The leadership can be permanent or rotated, according to committee's bylaws, but the charter of the committee should be upheld.

This committee has responsibility for managing all information coming into and going out of the organization. This includes automated and manual medical records, outcomes data, quality improvement teams, forms, telecommunications, telephones, and policies and procedures. This is a large task for one committee, but if there are only a few people making decisions, consistency and focus will be maintained.

# MANAGING THE PROJECT

Implementation management involves much more than putting a plan together and monitoring its progress. A good project leader understands the principles of time management and is skilled in running an effective meeting. Also, a major part of any implementation is the development and modification of the policies and procedures affected by the new system. A good project leader understands this and is able to provide the leadership to ensure that this is done properly.

# POLICIES AND PROCEDURES

There are many templates for writing policies and procedures. On the clinical side, it is common to see the use of *standard of care* and *standard of practice*. The standard of care states the policy and identifies the level of excellence that will be upheld. The standard of practice describes the methodology of how the organization will meet the standard of care. On the technical side, *policy* and *procedure* are the common headings. The policy describes what will be done, while the procedure explains how it will be accomplished.

The first step in developing policies and procedures is to identify the problem. Not every procedure requires a corresponding policy. In fact, one policy may have many procedures associated with it. For example, assume there has been a breach in confidentiality on one of the nursing units. Because this is an organizationwide issue, this problem will be addressed at a high level of administration. It would be useless and a waste of time to have every unit in the organization write its own confidentiality policy. The policies would differ in content and would be difficult to regulate. A subject like this one that must be handled consistently throughout the entire organization might be called a universal policy. Different procedures to implement the policy, however, may be written to cover the different circumstances within each department.

The method outlined in the following text has proven to be effective as a streamlined approach for identifying and documenting procedures that support written policies. With clinicians being educated in schools all over the globe, it is difficult, if not impossible, to guarantee that every care provider has been taught the same method for all the tasks they perform. Even though some procedures seem basic, it is important to write down methodology and have staff refer to it as often as needed.

Once the policy, or standard of care, has been identified, the procedures, or standards of practice, must be written out clearly. These specific steps can be both broadly and narrowly based. They define how care will be given in an organization. A broad category may be interpretation of legislation, such as the nursing practice act, and deciding how it applies to a given situation. A couple of examples of narrowly based procedures might be step-by-step instructions on inserting a catheter in a male patient on the urology unit, or from a systems perspective, the procedure for admitting a patient to the unit, using the system to record the data. Usually, procedures are documented because there has been a problem or inconsistency that caused a bad outcome in the past. Management decides on the approved method or process that will be used in the organization.

Procedures that describe what to do in the event of a system outage are called downtime procedures. Procedures that describe how to bring the system current, once the system is operational again, are called recovery procedures. These procedures discuss the seriousness of the outage—for example, minor, serious, critical—and outline the procedures that will be followed in the event of each type of outage. Figure 9–2 contains an example of downtime and recovery procedures.

The writing of policies and procedures should follow a prescribed methodology. The following elements are important:

---

### ANCILLARY DOWNTIME PROCEDURES

The following procedures apply to all ancillary departments except Lab and Radiology.

These procedures are to be followed during system downtime. Downtime may occur for a number of reasons. It may be planned or unplanned, and it may be localized (within a department), hospitalwide, or networkwide.

When the system goes down, you will be notified as to the nature and estimated duration of the interruption. You will also be told which downtime procedure to follow.

Depending on the circumstances, a downtime recovery team *may* be assembled to assist with the entry and statusing of orders, and synchronization of the system once the system returns to operation. The size and composition of this team will depend on the nature and extent of the system downtime.

A. Upon Notification
   1. All **Stat** orders will be telephoned from the floor. Stat orders will be followed by a written requisition.
   2. All **Routine** orders will be sent on a manual requisition form.
   3. Upon completion of the order, mark the order "Complete" and place the requisition in a designated stack to be used during system recovery.

B. Change of Shift
   1. Report to oncoming shift the status and disposition of all downtime requests.

C. Recovery
   1. The recovery team will update status of all orders entered into Order Entry during recovery according to the notes made on the order during downtime.
   2. Once all entries have been made, print a *complete and incomplete orders* report, and verify the report against the manual requisitions.

---

**Figure 9–2** Downtime and recovery procedures

- Identifying a problem
- Investigating all the issues
- Writing the draft procedures
- Approval from the decision-making group
- Submission to appropriate administration for approval
- Education of staff

There are three basic processes employed when looking at problems (Robertshaw et al., 1978). Ask the following questions to gain perspective:

- Defining the problem:
  — What is the problem?
  — What must be accomplished?
  — Who decides?
  — What is this organization's value system?
- Generating alternatives:
  — What are the alternatives?
  — How much will any alternative cost?
  — What will the effect be with each alternative?
- Evaluating the suggested alternatives:
  — Which alternative is best for this situation?
  — What are the factors affecting the worth of each alternative?

The problem must be assessed for risk to the patient, unit, organization, state, and so on. Using patient confidentiality as an example, investigation of the issue, research of the literature, review of the confidentiality policies of other health care organizations, and review by the legal department or risk management department could all prove helpful in determining what should be included in this policy. What group will write the draft policy? A confidentiality policy would have a major impact on the entire organization and should be addressed by an interdisciplinary group. We would recommend that the information management steering committee be the oversight group.

Once the policy statement has been defined, procedures follow. An investigation of how something should be done can take many avenues. Researching literature on the correct and current method of completing a task, asking about proper technique from a manufacturer, and surveying established nationally known experts on a subject all can be helpful. Once the organization is confident and comfortable with the facts, the procedure statement can be written.

Use a very simple writing format. The health care organization's logo and/or letter-head should be used for official documents. The following headings should be used:

• Subject
• Effective Date (and, if applicable, Previous Date)
• Administrative Approval
• Recommended by
• Standard of Care or Policy Statement (whatever is common in your organization)
• Standard of Practice or Procedure Statement

## Subject

The subject title should reflect the subject matter of the policy. Some health care organizations have indexed their policy and procedure manuals to reflect departments, or have outlined clinical versus administrative policy and procedure subjects. It is common to find policies alphabetized by the identified problem. It will work any way that is comfortable, as long as the method is easy to follow and remains consistent throughout the manual and the organization.

## Dates

The effective date or previous date is very important. The JCAHO regulations require that every policy in the organization be reviewed at least once every three years. There should be a process for continual renewal in place.

We have found that the following method works well, if it is maintained. It is recommended that every current and outdated policy be gathered, indexed, and assigned to the appropriate decision-making body. Policy review or writing becomes an agenda item for every meeting of each group. Each policy, hard copy or automated, is then placed in a tickler file. The group decides how often it will meet in a three-year period and divides the number of policies by the number of meetings.

The appropriate numbers of policies are assigned for investigation to each member of the group. This person reviews the policy, looking at current work flow, equipment, medications, titles, names, and so on, for timeliness and accuracy. At the assigned meeting, the policy is reviewed with the rest of the group. Each date the policy is reviewed should remain on the document.

## Approval

Administrative approval ensures that the policy and procedure has followed the appropriate path. Once the "recommended by" group has proposed a new or revised policy and procedure, someone in administration should review it and sign off on it. If the policy and procedure is placed in a manual or automated without an administrative signature, it is not official.

## Standard of Care or Policy Statement

The standard of care, or policy, is a statement that reflects what a patient or employee can expect from the organization. It is an overall statement that reflects the level of excellence that will be supported by the health care organization.

## Standard of Practice or Procedure Statement

The standard of practice, or procedure, outlines the steps that will be followed to ensure the standard of care will be fulfilled. This is the recipe to make the standard of care happen. This outline must be very clear and easy to understand. All employees, from the novice to the expert, should be able to follow the steps.

## Education

The last element of policy and procedure development is not something that appears in the policy or procedure itself. There are many ways of educating staff about a new policy or procedure. We have seen notebooks with new policies and procedures displayed to be read and initialed by staff. Once all staff members have initialed the new material, it is then cataloged in the manual. We have seen new policies and procedures hanging in the restroom. Initials, again, denote that these documents have been read. New policies and procedures are read at team or department meetings, and the sign-in sheets are used to document the staff's knowledge of the new material. Any method that works for the organization can be used. It is very important to educate staff and document it for each revision to policies and procedures.

---

### Case Scenario

For this example, let us assume the following scenario. Jack Smith is a physical therapist working the evening shift at Metro Hospital. His ex-wife, Jennifer Smith, is an inpatient on the psychiatric unit. At some time during Jennifer's stay, Jack enters Metro's HIS and reads Jennifer's entire medical record. He then tells several of his friends of his ex-wife's condition, and word spreads. The nurses on the psychiatric unit begin an investigation into this activity.

There are several issues to be considered here. Using the problem-solving process discussed earlier, let us answer each question and build consensus for a recommended punishment.

Given this situation, what is the problem? There has been a breach in confidential information. Jack did not have the need to know his ex-wife's medical diagnosis or treatment plan. There was no order for physical therapy, and even if there were, Jack would not have been the appropriate therapist.

What must be accomplished? The staff must be made aware of the seriousness of this act. This must not be allowed in the health care arena. Disciplinary action must be swift and aggressive. Education on this issue must be immediate and widespread.

Who decides? Due to the global nature of this case, the information management steering committee, top hospital administration, and human resources should be involved in the investigation and follow-through of this case.

What is this organization's value system? There is federal legislation and JCAHO regulations that dictate confidentiality and security of information in health care settings. The institution must protect every patient first and foremost. In this case, the employee, who should have been acting in the institution's behalf, was acting only for himself. The guidelines for disciplinary action are outlined in the human resources employee handbook. Top administration and the information steering committee must decide where this action falls along the guidelines.

What are the alternatives? Usually, disciplinary guidelines run from a first verbal warning to a first written warning with follow-up actions, second written warning with suspension of work days and follow-up actions, and then, finally, termination. Depending upon the injury, any of these steps can be skipped, resulting in immediate termination of the employee. Once the case has been investigated, administration must decide.

The other questions regarding how much the alternatives will cost and the effects of each alternative must be raised within this conversation. If Jack is allowed to remain as an active employee, what does this say about the organization's beliefs, not to mention its ability to uphold the federal and state laws concerning confidentiality?

The final questions in problem solving—which alternative is best for this situation, and what are the factors affecting the value of each alternative—must be answered to the satisfaction of everyone involved. A complete understanding of the current policy and future needs should be addressed.

Jack, being a physical therapist, should have access to clinical information because he could be called for patient care on any unit, so his computer access was appropriate. Many times access can be limited to the unit where the staff is physically located, but for flexibility, many hospitals have opted against this limitation. The investigation found that Jack, using his own sign-on code, could be traced to the exact terminal he used. The time he used it, the record he looked at, and the length of time he spent in that record could also be determined.

This case study demonstrates that a problem can involve several departments and have repercussions all across the continuum of care. Policy should cover all scenarios. If nursing is writing a policy on placing a catheter, every department in the hospital that may have the need to place a catheter should be involved with the decision-making process. Situations vary widely—from a rural clinical situation to OR environments, from pediatrics to geriatrics. All scenarios should be investigated and consensus reached to ensure that there is only one approved method for accomplishing a task.

## Comments on the Case Scenario

In reviewing the breach in confidentiality case, we would recommend that Jack be immediately terminated, due to national standards found through investigation of these kinds of criminal acts. It is within Jennifer's rights to pursue legal action against both Jack and *the health care organization* if she chooses to do so. When she entered the hospital for care, she signed an agreement for treatment; the hospital accepted her as a patient and, by doing so, assured her that they would maintain her medical records in a safe and confidential manner. This is an important part of the patient rights document. In addition to terminating Jack, written warnings should be given to all the "friends" to whom Jack had passed information. Confidentiality statements should be reviewed with every staff member and re-signed.

The current policy should be reviewed and revised to have the confidentiality statements signed yearly by every employee. Administration should use this case as an educational scenario and show strength and nontolerance for this activity.

Figure 9–3 is an example of a confidentiality policy for a health care organization.

## MEETINGS

Throughout the software application implementation, the team will be meeting to review progress and resolve problems. In addition, the information management

---

**General Hospital**
**123 Anywhere Street, Colorado Springs,**
**Colorado 80903**

**Subject:** Confidentiality—Patient
**Effective Date:** 3/98                                                        **Previous Date:** 6/95, 7/97

   **Administrative Approval:** John McMasters, CIO, 2/98
   **Recommended by:** Information Management Steering Committee
   **Standard of Care:** Any patient admitted to General Hospital can be assured that their medical information will be kept private and confidential.
   **Standard of Practice:** Each patient's rights as an individual will be respected, and any information, observations, communications, and records pertaining to the patient's care will be considered confidential.

- Each patient's right to privacy will be maintained at all times. Any information about the patient, location of the patient, their condition or physician's name, and so on will be considered confidential.
- All hospital personnel are personally accountable for their actions, on and off duty, and must exercise discretion when dealing with information—verbal, written, and automated—about patients in order to maintain the patient's right to confidentiality and protect persons who have no need to know such information.
- Printed materials that reveal any information about patients must not be posted in public places and will not be removed from the hospital premises.
- Access to patient records will be limited to medical staff, in-house professional and technical employees and students, and others specifically designated by the patient's physician or by administration.
- Health information system terminals will be used by personnel only for entering or retrieving information that is required or vital for the care of that patient.
- Any employee issued a sign-on code is responsible for protecting the security of that code.
- If there is any reason to believe a code has been compromised, it should be reported to the security officer in the IT department immediately. Any employee who abuses a sign-on code will be subject to appropriate disciplinary actions.
- For inquiries from the press, refer to Policy M-18, "News Media, Releasing Information to."

**Figure 9–3** Confidentiality policy

steering committee should be meeting periodically to review progress and provide guidance.

In most organizations, there is a general feeling that there are too many meetings that steal time from "productive" activities. If a meeting is not productive, it should not be held. Meetings are an integral part of any implementation. A lot of time is spent in meetings. For that reason, knowing how to get the most out of them is an important skill.

For our purpose, we will use the definition of a meeting as a structured situation where people work together in a give-and-take relationship to do one or more of the following (Gordon, 1981):

- Present
- Investigate
- Solve problems
- Expedite decisions
- Create new ideas and procedures
- Teach
- Train
- Evaluate

The groups holding these meetings are commonly called:

- Teams
- Committees
- Task forces
- Interest groups
- Focus groups
- Work groups

Who attends these meetings? There is the *leader,* or the person designated to run the meeting, and then there are the *members.* These are people who belong at the meetings because they can add expertise to the work that will be performed.

People come to meetings with skills that have been acquired in other situations. The following are the functions we commonly use in every meeting we attend:

- We experience activities and collect data about what is going on through thoughts, feelings, senses, actions, values, and will.
- We share this data with others by experiencing the same things at the same time.
- We combine this data to serve the purposes of the meeting.
- We apply generalizations to situations outside the meeting, bringing history and future to the present.
- We evaluate with questions.
- We experiment and take risks with new forms of behavior and beliefs.

Meetings can be a continuous series of agreements and disagreements. Gordon (1981) has identified several common methods of reaching a decision. He has attached names to each:

**The Slide.** This is a common, but often unnoticed, method. An idea is mentioned and is followed by more discussion until the entire group gravitates toward the initial idea.

**The Voting Booth.** This is known as "last-resort voting." It happens when differences among members cannot be resolved. These differences are generally understood by the members and tolerated, but each member must vote one way or the other.

**The Railroad.** This occurs when the leader or a member has a preconception or bias concerning an issue and insists that the rest of the members see it from his point of view. The person can maneuver the members by tabling the issue, volunteering to take care of it himself, or glossing over it by moving to another very demanding topic.

**The Hilltop.** The leader sees himself as having the final say on every decision. The members can argue all the issues, but the leader makes the final decision.

**The Perfect Circle.** This is the unanimous vote of support, which rarely happens. It is not necessary, for a functional team, to always come to total agreement on every issue.

**The Rainbow.** This is known as consensus. The key to consensus is flexibility. No one member insists upon maintaining a point of view at all costs. Instead, this point of view may be compared carefully with others and, if necessary, modified.

Consensus is the method of choice. Both the leader and the members emerge from the meeting with the feeling that they had a part in the decision-making process and, ultimately, in the outcome.

Every meeting has a purpose. There should be a predetermined outcome for each and every meeting. As an exercise, the next time you are sitting in a meeting, estimate the salary of each member, add up the total amount of money the organization is spending in the meeting, and judge whether the outcomes are worth the amount being spent. Too many meetings end without results, which is why we view many meetings as non-productive and a waste of valuable time.

## Lead

How can we make our meetings more meaningful and worth the time and cost? There are a number of techniques that can be easily learned. First of all, when you are the leader, lead. Here are some ideas:

- Arrive a few minutes early to make sure there are enough chairs. Arrange the furniture appropriately for your meeting.
- Always review the equipment. If a white board is needed and is not in the room, then a half hour may go by with someone trying to track one down.

- Make sure your meeting is scheduled. Always attempt to schedule consistently, for example, if this is a monthly meeting, always schedule for the first Monday of every month, at 3:00 P.M., in Meeting Room C.
- Mingle informally before the meeting starts. This shows you are approachable and want to be part of the team.
- Learn names and responsibilities of each of the members. Address them by their first names.
- Start the meeting on time.
- Introduce any visitors to the members. Explain why visitors are in attendance.
- Review announcements that affect the entire group.

Any latecomer should be neither rewarded nor punished, but invited to have a seat. Never review what you have already covered. If you need to catch someone up, attempt to do it during a break or after the meeting. It will not take too many meetings for the members to decide they need to be on time.

As the leader, set the ground rules of the meeting:

- Be clear about the tasks put before the members.
- Explain and clarify concepts to assist members in formulating thoughts and ideas surrounding the tasks.
- During each meeting, encourage members to speak only for themselves.
- Encourage members to both give and get from each meeting. Giving means to relate ideas, expertise, and comments concerning the topic. Getting means accepting othersí contributions to the theme and building upon those.
- Keep the discussion focused. Do not allow the topic to drift.
- Encourage members to be responsible for their actions and participation at each meeting.
- End every meeting with a clear statement of what was accomplished and what remains to be done.

## Agenda

Send out an agenda ahead of time. The agenda should include each topic, along with the time allotted to the topic and the responsible team member. If the organization has E-mail, make use of it. Always bring extra paper copies with you for those who forget their agenda. On the agenda, assign responsibilities and time limits to each agenda item.

The leader must facilitate the meeting. It is the leader's job to keep track of time frames, announce topics, and introduce members. If the item has a ten-minute time frame, it is the leader's job to remind members, after six minutes, that there are two minutes left for discussion and two minutes for the members to come to consensus on this issue, if it is needed. If it is a report that has been allotted ten minutes, after eight minutes, the leader should remind the speaker that the report should conclude within two minutes.

The leader must be forceful. The members of the group should be aware of the time frames allotted to them, and they should be expected to stick to these times. The meeting leader should move aggressively from topic to topic on the agenda. If there is no way a report will be completed or members will come to consensus within the time frame, the topic can be tabled until the next meeting, or some other agenda item can be tabled and this topic continued. Be strict about time.

## Remove Communication Roadblocks

One of the characteristics that make a good leader is to emphasize *listening.* Listening to all members and to the leader emphasizes the importance of each person participating in the meeting. Listening is probably the most important tool for effective communication. It is also the most neglected. People are generally more concerned with what they have to say than with listening to others (Grohar-Murray & DiCroce, 1992).

Learning to listen properly is a very powerful way to progress personally, as well as to ensure that your work team accomplishes all it possibly can. These are some simple steps to practice (Douglass & Douglass, 1992; Kieffer, 1988):

- Learn to focus. Many people believe they can do two or three things simultaneously. Information is internalized and remembered faster and better when your total attention is focused on one issue. When people continue to think about something else while someone is talking to them, simply nodding, "uh-huh" now and then, they are being disrespectful. Their actions tell the speaker that what the speaker is saying is not important. If it is worth listening to, devote your full attention to it. Filter out all other thoughts. Never bring other work with you to meetings.
- Learn to interpret what you hear. Any communication is more than just the words spoken. The better we know people, the greater the chance that we will understand what they are trying to say. Watch for nonverbal signals. Ask questions, and restate your understanding of what has been said. Two-way communication is an insurance policy for better understanding.
- Do not get so caught up in critiquing the delivery or the appearance of the speaker that you miss the message.
- Do not interrupt before the full message is delivered. Many times, if questions are taken during the presentation, it is difficult to get back the original focus intended.
- Do not yield to distractions, such as a telephone, beepers, a passerby, other thoughts, calendars, and so on.

The leader models behavior for the rest of the members. If the leader makes listening a high priority, then the members will likely follow suit.

## Time Management

If there are not enough activities to warrant meeting for an hour, then break when the agenda has been covered. Do not continue the meeting simply to fill the time. We are very good about using up every minute with small talk and irrelevant trivia. Use your time wisely.

Many health care organizations seem to be "meeting'd-to-death." A wise person will look at several meetings where the same people are attending each meeting and wonder, could we combine some of these? That does not mean changing three one-hour meetings into one three-hour meeting. It means looking at the agendas for overlapping subjects, cutting out chit-chat, sticking to valuable agenda items, maintaining time frames, and getting real work accomplished. Here are some tips on managing time (Douglass & Douglass, 1992):

- Take time to write down and clarify your goals and expectations. There may be an attempt to focus on several projects, often trying to do everything at once. The usual outcome results in losing the ability to do anything at all.
- Think things through before agreeing to take on another project. Do not be too quick to be agreeable. Consider the ability of others to get the project done. Can you delegate some of the work? How committed are you currently? Can one or more of your current projects wait until you complete this new one? Ask yourself, can I do a good job on all my assignments?
- Learn to make realistic time estimates. We often fail to realize how long things take, thus multiplying problems later. Compromise on dates whenever possible. Ask why a date has been issued. Are there other factors associated with it that are waiting until you get your part of the project accomplished?
- Be patient with others. Do not yell or raise your voice. Start earlier and give people more lead time. Be slow to add more to an already full plate.
- Interrupt others less. Do not interrupt others who are working if the question can wait.
- Pay attention when people talk to you. Look at them. Be present for them.
- Compete less and cooperate more. Learn to work with others, even difficult ones. You can accomplish far more than you could ever accomplish alone.
- Slow down a little. Do not demand so much of yourself and others. Realize that relaxing is a crucial part of good time management. It refreshes you and helps you gain new perspective.

- Take yourself a little less seriously. Most things are not as critical as you may think. Ask yourself, "Will this matter in five years?" Learn to laugh at yourself.
- Finish what you start before jumping to something else. Try to complete at least one task before moving on to yet another crisis.
- Focus on developing an on-time habit. Being late is perceived as being lazy. Change your ways.
- Set aside ten minutes a day for simple planning. Plan at the same time every day. Review what you have accomplished today, and plan where you will start tomorrow.
- Once a team has developed a plan, stick to it. Do not be tempted to take off in another direction. The team is counting on every member following the initial plan.
- Try to develop more routines in your life. It is freeing, rather than confining, because you are confident you will get the important major tasks accomplished.
- Curb your socializing time. When you are at work, remain focused on work. If you socialize during your work hours, the work still remains, causing overtime and working late.
- Stop procrastinating. Break large jobs down into smaller pieces and focus on one piece at a time.
- Learn that positive, planned change will make your life better. Change does not have to be bad or frightening. Different can be exciting.
- Be more assertive. Learn to say no more often, without an excuse attached.

Remember that people are more important than procedures. Regardless of the situation, we can all learn to be good time managers and excellent team players.

## Meeting Minutes

It is important to document meetings correctly. Save time and improve clarity by using an easy format. Attendance should be the first item of business. This can be as easy as a sign-in sheet being passed around. Have the attendees print both their names and their titles. The JCAHO regulations encourage interdisciplinary representation on decision-making committees. It is easy to prove interdisciplinary representation if titles are on the sign-in sheet. If roll is to be called, have a master copy of the roll call and include the titles of members.

The following brief format for meeting minutes is very effective:

- Issue
- Discussion
- Action/resolution

- Any follow-up needed
  — Assign responsibility
  — Time frames for follow-up

## Issue

A simple word or description that matches the agenda item identifies the topic for discussion. A list of all outstanding issues should be kept and monitored to ensure that nothing "falls through the cracks."

Create a simple issues list database for the software application implementation project. Every team, from the smallest work group to the information management steering committee, should maintain an issues list. When an issue is raised in one of these meetings and can not be resolved before the meeting adjourns, add the issue to the issues list. For each issue, document the following:

- A brief description of the issue
- The party responsible for researching and presenting a recommendation for resolution of the issue
- The date the issue is added to the list
- The target date for resolution of the issue
- The date the issue is actually resolved
- Other parties/departments that may be impacted by the issue
- A brief description of the resolution

A simple database is easy to build, using one of the popular microcomputer-based database management systems. By managing the issues list through one of these tools, it is easy to sort and print the issues for additions to the meeting agenda. A sort by "responsible party" will print all the issues by individual team member. A sort by "target date" will produce the issues that are scheduled for resolution. Figure 9–4 displays an issue printed in an issues list format.

## Discussion

In documenting discussion, most of time it is not important that "Sue said," "Bob replied," "Joe commented." It is important to document the essence of the conversation, report, or issue. One or two sentences should be enough to describe the actual conversation. Put more than that in the minutes only if it is absolutely needed.

## Action/Resolution

The action related to the issue may be ongoing. The resolution will be the conclusion of an issue. Either of these may be appropriate for different topics during the meeting.

| | Resolution Affects | Assigned To | Date Added to List | Resolution Target Date | Date Resolved |
|---|---|---|---|---|---|
| Issue: How will Orders and Results be handled for inpatients transferred to OR?<br><br>Resolution: Diet orders will be suspended for all inpatients sent to OR. All clinical orders will remain active. The Results will be routed to OR and Recovery until the patient is returned to the Unit. See Policy # 1234. | Nursing Ancillaries OR | MPP | 08/01/97 | 08/20/97 | 08/20/97 |
| Issue:<br><br>Resolution: | | | | | |

**Figure 9–4** Issues list

The important thing is that the disposition of every relevant issue be documented. If an action is ongoing, place it immediately on the issues list and on the agenda as an item for follow-up. If there is resolution, then reflect the conclusion and move on.

## *Assigning Responsibility and Follow-up*

Many times, topics are either continuous or take more than one meeting to complete. Follow-up allows the subject to continue, but not get lost along the way. Always include instructions regarding the responsible party and the follow-up required, for example, "Larry Jones will interview three hospitals of like size and environment to gather information on order-entry procedures."

Either the secretary or the leader of the group should keep all minutes and agendas as a history of the committee's activities. A three-ring binder is useful for this purpose, as pages can be easily added. It is not uncommon, during long implementations, to reach decisions that are later questioned. It is very useful to have a complete history of activities.

# MONITORING THE PROJECT

Using the implementation plan and the issue list, the team leader should review the status of the project on a weekly basis. In a team meeting, each member can provide an update of his progress on the specific tasks he has been assigned. If progress is expressed in terms of percent complete, it is a minor task to update the project-scheduling tool. The scheduling tool will automatically update the entire project.

Gantt charts can be produced to report to the steering committee and other interested parties. Gantt charts are recommended because they communicate a lot of information in an efficient pictorial format. Another advantage to using the project-scheduling tool, in the Gantt format as a reporting tool, is that groups of activities can be expanded or contracted to focus on specific areas of the plan or to customize the presentation to the audience. You may want full detail for team meetings and less detail for the steering committee and other groups.

As situations change, change the plan. Never allow the project to get out of sync with the plan. Through judicious maintenance of the project plan and close attention to the issues list, even the largest system implementation can be kept under control. The biggest enemy of a system implementation is surprise. The best way to avoid surprises is to be aware of the progress, or lack thereof, of the project activities and the issues that arise around them.

# PROJECT MANAGEMENT TOOLS

The following is a list of some of the project management programs available on the market. Many of these can be run on a standard microcomputer:

- InstaPlan-EMS, Micro Planning International
- Microsoft Project for Windows, Microsoft Corporation
- Project Workbench
- Harvard Project, Software Publishing
- Microman, POC-IT
- Ca Superproject, Computer Associates
- Timeline, Sysmantic Corporation
- Project Director, adRem Technologies, Inc.
- Project Scheduler, Scitor Corporation
- SureTrak Project Scheduler, Primavera

# REFERENCES

Douglass, M. E., & Douglass, D. N. (1992). *Time management for teams.* New York: American Management Association.

Gordon, M. (1981). *Making meetings more productive.* New York: Sterling.

Grohar-Murray, M. E., & DiCroce, H. R. (1992). *Leadership and management in nursing.* Norwalk, CT: Appleton & Lange.

Hradesky, J. L. (1998). *Productivity & quality improvement: A practical guide to implementing statistical process control.* New York: McGraw-Hill.

Kieffer, G. D. (1988). *The strategy of meetings.* New York: Simon & Schuster.

Robertshaw, J., Mecca, S. J., & Rerick, M. N. (1978). *Problem solving: A systems approach.* New York: Petrocelli.

# CHAPTER

# Security and Confidentiality Issues

Before we can protect something, we must identify it and place a value on it. Information is intangible. Although we know what it is, we cannot really see it or touch it. So, we usually refer to it as reports, writings, bits, bites, numbers, and so on. It is difficult to identify and value. The implied worth of a piece of information is based on (1) its cost to produce or replace, (2) potential effects of its exposure or loss to the business, or (3) legal effects of loss (Schweitzer, 1987).

Every health care organization has a responsibility to itself, to its patients, and to the community at large to have good control of its information systems. Because the internal workings of a health care organization rely on accurate and timely data and information, personal data about employees and patients must be kept safe and confidential. A corporate security plan is important to an organization, with much of the corporation's competitive edge depending on controlling the information available to it (Fites & Kratz, 1993).

We will use the term *confidentiality* to refer to the trust placed in individuals to whom information is disclosed that the privacy of the information will be respected and the information will be used only for the purpose for which it was disclosed. *Security* will be defined as the protection of the information from accidental or intentional access by unauthorized people, from unauthorized modification, and from unauthorized accidental or intentional destruction (Ball & Hannah, 1984).

Security policies must be explicit and well defined. The intent of a security policy is to delineate what is expected of the organization concerning information systems security (Burn & Caldwell, 1990). These policies normally cover expected behavior, control of access to information, control of use and dissemination of information, a mandate that systems should remain available, and a plan for the business continuity in the event of a widespread disaster.

The term *risk management* will be used to describe the ideas, models, methods, and techniques used to control the risk. Fites and Kratz (1993) suggest that when considering the risk to anything, one must:

- Identify risk prevention, reduction, assignment, and acceptance.
- Order or rank internal versus external, accidental versus intentional, modification versus disclosure, dishonest versus disgruntled, and so on.
- Contrast effective versus efficient.
- Contrast hazard, vulnerability, exposure, and risk.
- Contrast probability and rate of occurrence.
- Contrast quantitative versus qualitative risk analysis.
- Rank hazards by damage or rate of occurrence, for example, fire versus water, error versus malice, and so on.
- Rank protective measures by effectiveness or efficiency, for example, supervision versus access control.
- Contrast acceptance versus assignment.
- Apply principles of cost-benefit analysis.
- Apply automated risk analysis systems.

The Joint Commission on Accreditation of Healthcare Organizations (JCAHO) has created an entire standard concerned with confidentiality and security issues. It is found as Information Management Standard IM.2. It covers three main areas of concern:

IM. 2.1—The hospital determines appropriate levels of security and confidentiality for data and information.

IM 2.2—Collection, storage, and retrieval systems are designed to allow timely and easy use of data and information without compromising its security and confidentiality.

IM 2.3—Records and information are protected against loss, destruction, tampering, and unauthorized access or use. (JCAHO, 1998)

This is the federal mandate that provides opportunities to health care organizations to define confidentiality, provide security, and maintain and protect their information.

Protection in a health care organization must be the integration of various security elements occurring all at once. We will look at the physical plant first, beginning with the identification of assets: what needs to be protected? Usually these four physical components emerge:

1. Facility: building, rooms, workspace, and backup storage area
2. Support: air conditioning, fire systems, electricity, communications, water, fuel supplies, power, and so on
3. Computer components: hardware such as CPUs, printers, disk drivers, and terminals; desks, chairs, and office furniture; office equipment; telephones; reference books; files; ergonomic aids; and personal objects
4. Supplies and materials: tapes, disks, paper supplies, waste material, and so on

Facility security involves the use of access controls, double doors, and alarms to ensure the safety of the computer, the computer room, and the computer operators, thereby protecting the information contained in the computers. Physical security ensures the ability of continuing information services to the organization.

## RISK ASSESSMENT

When doing a risk assessment of the physical location and construction of the building, consider where the building is, how it is built, and whether there are protection elements in place. Consider the vulnerability to crime, riots, or demonstrations. Are there issues with protection of the staff leaving after hours or entering the building in the middle of the night? Is the parking structure or parking lot well lit, fenced in, or monitored? How close is the building to police and fire protection?

Are there adjacent buildings and/or businesses nearby? What kind of work do they do? Could there be explosives, fire hazards, chemical spills, or radiation hazards right next door? Is the adjacent building attached to your building in any way? If so, is the security strong enough to keep intruders out? It is recommended that a complete disaster recovery and business resumption plan be written, activated, and reviewed on an annual basis.

Computers need electrical power to work. Most computers are sensitive to "dirty power." The power supply conditions should be monitored. Power supplies should not be shared with other needs in the building. There are automatic devices available that keep record of electrical usage and any surges that occur. Using surge protectors on every PC may be all that is needed to keep electrical supply even.

Static is another risk of nature. Particularly in cold climates, people generate static electricity just by moving around in a normal manner. When the humidity is low, sparks are common, and a spark can ruin a computer chip or scramble data on a diskette. Regulating humidity in the environment minimizes static. Antistatic mats under chairs and machines and antistatic carpeting, as well as antistatic sprays, can help in a computer environment (Fites & Kratz, 1993).

When mainframe architecture was common, health care organizations usually had one room that housed a huge mainframe computer. This room met all the criteria, such as a special air-conditioning system, automatic humidity and temperature monitoring equipment, fire controls, isolated power supply, and locked doors. The storage area for the tape backups was treated in much the same manner. With the advent of client-server technology, servers are placed almost everywhere without much thought to security, air conditioning, and power or fire controls. Policy should reflect the thought process concerning these issues with each server placed outside a computer room in the health care environment (Bennatan, 1995).

## TRAINING

Training the staff to use backup tapes on a regular basis is important. These tapes should be stored in a locked, fireproof area and checked periodically to verify the information on them. Is the backup procedure really working? There have been incidences where a backup tape has been needed but, when restored, did not have any information on it at all. One can only imagine the frustration for the user, knowing the hours that had been spent doing backups, when faced with the need for the backup, only to find that the restored procedure had not worked. Test the backup and restore procedures. Loss of information residing on individual PCs, depending on the employees' responsibilities, could have major impact on the organization if reports or projects are lost to acts of God, hard drive crashes, or vandalism.

The security of information policy should include preventative measures for computer viruses. Downloading infected diskettes onto the health care organization's network or individual PCs transmits most viruses. Prevention comes from two main sources:

1. Protection
2. Detection

Using only trusted software sources, and scanning any "at-risk" diskette, are protective measures. Checking and scanning PCs periodically are detective controls. Common factors included in this policy would be:

• Accept diskettes and programs only from trusted sources.
• Scan all files and diskettes for viruses. Use more than one scanning program.
• Make backup copies of clean diskettes, store originals for safekeeping, and operate from the copies.
• Never boot the computer from a diskette.
• Install a memory-scanning tool on each PC.

Since new viruses are spreading daily, continuous efforts are needed to protect against viruses (Fites & Kratz, 1993).

## STAFF PROTECTION

The next level of concern is the staff. Once you have provided a safe environment, the employees who work in the facility must be protected, as well as the data and information they produce and use daily. This will be accomplished by putting several security measures in place.

People, or personnel, are the ones who make an organization successful. It is also people who protect or try to harm the organization. Fites & Kratz (1993) report that eighty-five percent of all people are strictly honest; they would not commit a crime regardless of temptation and opportunity. Of the other fifteen percent, perhaps five percent would engage in a dishonest act if they believed there was no chance of getting caught, another five percent might risk a small chance, and the final five percent might try, even if there were a fifty-fifty chance of being caught. The potential or actually dishonest people are the security concerns.

This study goes on to say that criminal behavior involves three basic elements:

1. Dishonesty
2. Opportunity
3. Motive

If there is no reason to do something (motive), there is little risk. If there is no opportunity to do something, there is little risk. If the person is one of the eighty-five percent that are honest, there is little risk. The goal for the health care organization is to reduce work-related incentives for people to cause trouble. Since there is life outside the workplace (large debts, espionage, gambling problems, and other nonwork activities), other controls must be reviewed.

Employee selection is the first step in prevention. It is imperative to have an accurate job description. It wastes time for the applicants and the management to review resumes and go through interviews if the job is not properly defined and communicated. Once the job is posted, there are a few basic security tools to aid in the selection of an honest employee:

- Application forms
- Permissions for investigations
- Reference and document checks
- Security clearances and citizenship

All applicants should be required to fill out an application before being interviewed. The intent of using an application is to put relevant information into the same format. While information systems positions are very different from nursing positions, general background information is still necessary. Some suggested components of an application form are: [*You may want to review the form your health care organization uses, to ensure these areas of information are covered.*]

- Name: first, last, middle, nicknames, maiden names
- Was the name ever legally changed? If so, when and where, and what was the previous name?
- Date and place born
- Current address and previous addresses *(for at least the last ten years)*
- Telephone number, beeper number, fax number, E-mail address
- Employment history, most recent jobs first (all times since leaving high school must be accounted for, including periods of unemployment; gaps are significant warning signals)
- Company name, address, previous bosses' names and titles
- Date hired and terminated, and reason for leaving
- Job title and nature of the job; salary or wage
- Education: names of schools, dates attended, field of study, highest degree obtained
- Health considerations relevant to job performance
- Credit references
- Personal references (three names, addresses, and telephone numbers of people the applicant has known longer than two years—nonrelatives)
- Criminal record, if any

At the bottom of the application form, include a paragraph that makes the applicant aware that you expect true answers:

I attest that the information provided above is true and complete to the best of my knowledge and belief. I understand that falsification or misrepresentation of any data provided in this application may be grounds for refusing or terminating employment. I authorize (company name) to check any data provided.

Signed: _____

Date: _____

The final point made in the study concerning the interview process is a note to management: *check everything*. It has been estimated that between ten and thirty percent of resumes contain misrepresentations or actual falsehoods (Fites & Kratz, 1993). Specific things to watch for include:

- Gaps in employment history—ask about each, as this is the most common area of misrepresentation
- Frequent job moves
- Unusual previous salaries
- Unusual educational background for previous jobs
- Name changes (check under all names)
- Confirm the following:
  — References: if you can not reach someone, ask the applicant for another name and number
  — Previous employment
  — Transcripts
  — Professional certificates
  — Credit record (large debts may indicate risk)
  — Criminal record

Although all the information discussed here is common knowledge, many times steps in the process are bypassed, due to the urgency to get a position filled. Even with all the precautions taken to hire the right person, none of these can guarantee a honest person. The organization must use other methods in the attempt to keep the information secure.

The use of employee swipe cards attempts to ensure the person entering the building is an employee. Policy should reflect the surrendering of these cards upon termination of employment and should explain the process for getting a new card if an employee's card is lost or stolen. The address of the organization should be printed on the back of the card, guaranteeing postage if someone finds it and drops it in the mail. Any lost cards should be reported to security immediately. A listing of all issued swipe cards should be maintained.

Some other common options for an employee entering a building are keypad code devices, retina scanners, security cameras, and live guards. None of these methods are without problems. Keypads use universal codes; therefore, many people are aware of the code and have access. It is a widely accepted practice to change these universal codes at agreed-upon time frames. Some organizations are comfortable with changing them every thirty days; some will change them every six months; and others may fall anywhere in between. With the numbers of employees entering and leaving the health care organizations today, and an increase in vandalism and sabotage against employers, this becomes necessary for the safety of everyone and all the equipment. Whenever a code is changed, it is common for staff to write it down somewhere as a reminder, which is precisely the wrong thing to do. Policy should cover the sharing of codes between staff members and the documentation of codes.

Retina scanners have been used for only the last couple of years, but they have been blamed for serious eye infections, caused by many employees using the same reader with no sanitation means between uses. Employees sometimes feel uncomfortable with this procedure.

The use of live security guards or security cameras discourages the sharing of codes and meets sanitary guidelines, but around-the-clock security is expensive. Swipe cards are commonly used (Schweitzer, 1987).

Name tags with pictures are frequently used in clinical areas, as well as in the information services area. These, like the swipe cards, should be laminated to decrease the chance of altering pictures and names. Again, policy should reflect the surrendering of the name badge upon termination of employment. All sales representatives should be required to sign in on a log sheet and be issued a labeled badge for admittance.

## PATIENT CONFIDENTIALITY

In patient care areas, there should not be any patient-identifying information outside the rooms. This is a safety, confidentiality, and privacy issue. The days of name tags beside the doors and I/O sheets with names on them are gone. Visitors should ask at the desk for the room number of a family member or friend, and they may be asked for identification. If the patient wishes to be a "silent" patient, or one whose name is kept confidential, then this wish must be respected by the health care organization.

Overhead paging of patients or family members should be avoided. The use of "white boards," commonly found in rehabilitation areas, birth centers, and emergency rooms, should have patient initials only on them or be placed out of view of the public. There is no need for the public to know how many centimeters a patient is dilated, or what tests are being run on the trauma victim in room 3, or what the rehabilitation schedule for Mr. Jones is on Friday. Privacy of information is vitally important. Always put yourself in the patient's place and ask, "Would I want anyone walking by to know that information about me?" If it appears to be public information in the hospital, does that make it appropriate public information for the local church group, or the grocery store aisle, or the hometown newspaper?

## PATIENT DATA

Security of patient data and information is of utmost importance. When a patient enters a health care organization, the patient signs an agreement for treatment. As a part of the admission, the hospital has the responsibility to not only treat that patient, but also to keep records of the treatment provided and the response to that treatment from the patient. This is called the medical record. Many specialists and professionals write and record observations in a patient's chart. The medical record can be manual or automated. It is most common today to have a mixture of both. Both the manual and automated portions must be covered by the same security and confidentiality measures.

Nationwide health care organizations are expanding into community clinics, outlying home care, and visiting nurse agencies. They are acquiring physician practices and setting up hospice situations and long-term care facilities. In each of these health care entities, a medical record is kept. If the hospital is the parent organization, the policy and procedures for keeping the medical record fall to the hospital. The organization's entire continuum of care must maintain the same security and confidentiality for all its medical records.

## MEDICAL RECORD

There may be some question about who can write in the medical record. Policy, usually found in the medical staff rules and regulation manual, should be in place to define who, how, and where staff can document care. The use of electronic signatures, the use of rubber stamps for signatures, and even the color of ink in ballpoint pens should be covered.

## CONFIDENTIALITY STATEMENTS

For all employees, volunteers, physician office staff, interpreters, students, transcriptionists, and anyone else who has access to confidential patient information, it is recommended that a confidentiality statement be discussed and signed. This process usually begins at the time of hiring, just after computer training has been completed and the new employee's code has been given to him. It is recommended that a review of the confidentiality and security policy and a signing of a new confidentiality statement become a yearly process. This review increases awareness throughout the health care community of the importance of keeping patient information confidential.

## CONFIDENTIALITY AND SECURITY MEASURES

Ongoing campaigns that cover not only automated information, but all kinds of information that moves around the health care organization, should be considered. Processes to review include:

Telephone conversations: how much personal information is routinely given out to callers

Faxed information: who has access to the fax machine on the other end

Laptops: many home care nurses are using laptops to gather information on their clients, and these same laptops are being used by the nurses' children to do homework in the evening

Casual conversations in the lunch room, hallways, or elevators: one is often unaware of other listeners

The picking up and delivering of patient charts in open chart racks around the hospital and leaving them unattended

There may be many other incidents of failure to keep information secure in the health care organization, but with heightened awareness, some of these will disappear (Schweitzer, 1987).

There are new inventions that we consider commonplace in today's technology that need special attention. These include fax machines, computer terminals, both on the units and at the bedside, and photocopying machines. We will look closer at each one.

## Fax Machines

The fax machine allows printed information to travel across telephone lines very quickly. In the health care organization, we may use this technology to gain access to test results rapidly, to order supplies easily, or to send out notification about an important event. This machine is useful in many ways. But because this technology uses telephone lines to move information, it also uses telephone numbers as addresses. As telephone users, we know how easy it is to dial a wrong number. This same phenomenon occurs with fax machines. Are we ever sure of who will receive this faxed material and have access to the confidential information it may contain? It is recommended that a fax cover sheet with a disclaimer describing the possibility of confidential information be used in all cases. Although a disclaimer will not stop receivers from looking at the information, it will put them on notice that it is not appropriate.

Another practice worthy of consideration is the quarterly testing of fax numbers your department commonly uses. Simply send out a fax cover sheet with instructions to fill out the identifying information questions and fax it back. Keep records of changes and of sheets that are not returned. Check to see if these numbers are still accurate or if the businesses are still viable. Every department in the organization should do this.

## Computer Terminals

Computer terminals are seen frequently on the nursing units. Computers bring patient information to workers' fingertips in a timely and efficient manner. If the nursing staff or physicians can get to the information fast and from many different locations, then decisions can be made faster and care can be delivered more quickly. Steps and time are saved. The workers have a need to know this information. We, as patients, want the staff to know. The public does not have a need to know. Health care organizations must be concerned about the placement of computer terminals in patient rooms, community lobbies, and patient care hallways. Many hospitals were built well before the computer age, and the physical location of terminals can present major problems. Fire codes and other regulations increase the creativity used in many cases. Behind all these decisions, confidentiality and security of information, and of the terminals themselves, must be a driving factor.

If there were a perfect choice for placement of computer screens, the ideal would be placement where the staff would have access, but no one else. Many times terminals must be placed in old closets, cubbyholes, and hallways. This makes terminal placements in hallways, lobbies, and patient rooms somewhat less than perfect. Other measures must be used to keep voyeurs and hackers out.

### Computer Passwords

In essence, security is a tradeoff for access. More access implies a lower level of security. Each organization must choose the level of exposure consistent with its desired ease of access (Fites & Kratz, 1993). Two-tiered user passwords are provided, usually using the first initial and last name of the user as the initial identification, and then a secret combination of several letters and/or numbers as the second layer of the code. Policy should discourage users from sharing or writing down their code. It should encourage users to select uncommon codes. It is not wise to use the names of children, spouses, or pets, or to use addresses or social security numbers (Mikuleky & Ledford, 1987). These codes are easy to trace, and a hacker can easily gain access with very little information. The ideal code is a combination of both numbers and letters, but this is also the most difficult to remember, especially when the software forces the user to change this secret code frequently.

### Employee Termination

When reviewing all the computer code issues, review the process for canceling the code of a discharged employee. If any employee is found to have falsified or misrepresented information when hired, the employee should be terminated. Employees guilty of serious violations of company policy regarding security and controls should be terminated. Employees guilty of unlawful acts should be prosecuted as well as terminated. Such action should be highly visible to employees, demonstrating that management takes security very seriously. Any termination should trigger certain steps, including:

• All company identification, including badges, IDs, business cards, and business-related materials, should be collected.
• All keys and swipe cards should be collected.
• All relevant locks, codes, passwords, and access codes must be changed immediately.
• Other members of the staff should be informed of the termination.

In many health care organizations, the human resource department will issue a list of terminated employees once each week. This may not be often enough. It is common in information systems departments to have security escort a discharged or laid off employee out the door. The IT employee may have the knowledge and skill to harm information in a manner that could take months to repair. There should be a process in place, given certain circumstances, to delete codes immediately, without having to wait several days for a list to be generated.

### Screen Savers

Another preventative option, usually found within the software, is the capability to activate a blackout screen or a screen saver. The terminal screen will black out after a predetermined amount of time has passed without usage. There are several things to be aware of, for example, some blackout curtains remain black until the mouse is moved or a key is struck, and then the screen will return to the last place the user was. While this is convenient for the user, it is also too convenient for the hacker. The other option is to have the screen black out and sign off the user and the terminal. While this option is more inconvenient for the health care staff, it is much more appropriate when confidentiality and security are priorities. It is difficult to defend against a hacker when you are saving a place within the system that he can access with only the slightest movement of the mouse or the strike of one key.

## Photocopying Machines

The last machine that needs comment is the photocopying machine. Again, with precious little space in hospitals, many times photocopying machines are placed in public corridors or spaces with no doors. Health care workers often photocopy confidential information. There are many times users pick up the copy and leave the original in the machine. It is advisable to use signs to remind users to take the originals.

## Waste Paper

While speaking of machines, each of these three machines produces waste paper. The printouts from a printer and the wasted copies from the copy machine and fax machine must be disposed of properly. Paper shredders are useful for this purpose, but they can be expensive if there is only a small amount of paper to shred. It is recommended that closed, labeled containers be used for disposal of confidential information. These containers must have the ability to be emptied, but they should not be made so that it is easy for someone to reach in and pull out documents. Something as simple as a clearly labeled plastic box with a slit cut in the cover can be used. This is a inexpensive way to meet this requirement.

## Treatment Documents

While the machines generate confidential documents, health care staff use these documents in their everyday work. Nurses carry around notes on several patients so they know what tasks, medications, exercises, and appointments the patients may need. What happens to these pieces of paper at the end of the shift? They *should* be disposed of properly while the nurse is still at the hospital. What often happens is, the nurse puts them in her pocket and takes them home. These notes contain confidential information; once the nurse is at home, they should be shredded or burned so as not to end up in the landfill. Staff members who carry notes should be encouraged to leave all documentation at the hospital.

## Vendors

Once confidential information is disposed of properly, it is the hospital's responsibility to contract with a reputable disposal company that will take proper care of it. The contract with this company should include a signed confidentiality statement.

## Physician Offices

It is common today for hospitals to have several physician offices contracting with the hospital. The question must be raised, whose information is it anyway? The office staffs are employees of the physician's; therefore, the physicians are responsible for the security of the information the hospital shares with their offices. It is recommended that all physician office staff sign the same confidentiality statement used by the hospital employees. Encourage the physicians to use the same policies and procedures that are being supported in the hospital.

## Paging

An uncomfortable situation occurred in a very large, well-known specialty hospital. In the intensive care area, family members were made comfortable in a large waiting area. There was coffee service, pillows and blankets, many games, and televisions around the room to accommodate the families and visitors. This was all very nice. It was disturbing, however, that the volunteers used overhead speakers to call out family names for telephone calls and physician calls. If numbers or vibrating beepers had been distributed, as they are in the restaurant business, the overhead paging would not have been necessary. With other means available, names should not be used.

## Media

Other media activities should be addressed as well. Even today, there are still hospitals that allow patient names and room numbers to be published in the hometown newspaper. Although this is probably done in good faith, the information is no one's business, and this is a breech of confidentiality. The names of newborns should be published only with signed letters of disclosure. While we take much of this for granted, we need to review our procedures and policies to make certain that the health care organization is taking every precaution to ensure the privacy, confidentiality, and security of patient information.

## Remote Computer Access

It is common for physicians and others to have dial-in access to the health care organization's systems. This affords the convenience of being at home or at the office and having the ability to write orders, review results, or make notes on the patient electronic medical record. Security measures must be in place to guarantee that it is the physician or other appropriate staff only entering the record. Many times passwords or dial-back procedures are used. All members of the office staff and the family members of the physician should know the policy concerning the use of the computer. Care must be taken to keep confidential information secure, while giving physicians and staff the access (Ball & Hannah, 1984).

## Internet Access

Last, but certainly not least, there is the question about Internet access. While the Internet is a huge resource for medical journals and published articles, there are also abuses happening in the health care organization. The first question should always be, what is the staff using the Internet for? Is it entertainment for the on-call doctor who cannot sleep in the middle of the night, or will it substitute for an on-site library? Policy should reflect appropriate uses and amount of time permitted.

Transferring information over the Internet is yet another topic for caution. Never send patient information via E-mail. The industry is attempting to build "firewalls" to ensure confidentiality. Some health care organizations are sending patient information across the

Internet, but only after building adequate firewalls and encryption techniques. Use extreme caution when doing this. Check out the stability and security very carefully.

Security and confidentiality demand a very complicated and interdisciplinary effort. Strict policy should be in place and maintained. Frequent testing of safeguards will ensure the reliability of the systems.

# REFERENCES

Ball, M. J., & Hannah, K. J. (1984). *Using computers in nursing.* Reston, VA: Reston Publishing Co.

Bennatan, E. M. (1995). *On time, within budget software project management practices and techniques* (2nd ed.). New York: Wiley.

Burn, J., & Caldwell, E. (1990). *Management of information systems technology.* Chippenham, Wiltshire, England: Antony Rowe.

Fites, P. E., & Kratz, M. P. (1993). *Information systems security.* New York: Van Norstrand Reinhold.

Joint Commission on Accreditation of Healthcare Organizations. (1998). *Comprehensive accreditation manual for hospitals.* Oakbrook Terrance, IL: Author.

Mikuleky, M. P., & Ledford, C. (1987). *Computer in nursing.* Menlo Park: Addison-Wesley.

National Bureau of Standards. (1975, May 30). *Computer security guidelines for implementing the Privacy Act of 1974* (FIPS-PUB-41). Springfield, VA: U.S. Department of Commerce.

Schweitzer, J. A. (1987). *Computers, business, and security.* Boston: Butterworths.

# CHAPTER

# Ergonomics

The electronic office has dramatically changed the way we do business. It has enhanced our ability to gather and exchange information without ever leaving our chair. We find documents in files on the computer, not in a file cabinet. We can print hard copies on a printer, with no typing or photocopying. And it has changed how we work.

People spend long hours in front of a computer screen, performing repetitive tasks. They work in noisy, poorly lit offices, seated in a fixed position on chairs and at desks meant for other tasks (Franchi & Fleck, 1994). For years, people pecked away at typewriters with few complaints of painful symptoms. Now computer users are experiencing large numbers of cumulative trauma injuries. These injuries are frequent because we no longer have to move a manual carriage return or stretch to insert paper into or remove paper from the typewriter. We communicate via E-mail and never have to reach to pick up a telephone. We have become stationary. We need to move.

Ergonomics is the "science of adapting working conditions to suit the individual's physical capacities and comfort" (Phair, 1995). A couple decades ago, employers ignored this concept, but today, *ergonomics* is a buzzword around the office. In the future, work areas will be ergonomically correct for all workers. This change is the result of an enormous increase in the frequency of painful injuries from cumulative trauma and in the costs associated with these injuries.

The workers' compensation system was enacted in the United States in 1908. Today, this insurance coverage is required by state laws, whether a business has one employee or hundreds (Anchin, 1996). The laws were originally designed to compensate workers for acute traumatic injuries occurring on the job. It quickly became apparent that it was less costly for the employers to make the workplace safer than to compensate injured workers (Rademaker, 1992). As time has passed, the initial concept has been expanded to include illness and injuries related to the workplace environment. The definitions of *illness* and *trauma* overlap. The first cases to be addressed were for spinal column claims. The spinal claims quickly expanded to include muscles and tendons of the upper and lower back. Due to the delicate connection of all these parts of the body, the workers' compensation definition was changed so as not to focus directly on a specific part of the body, but on the reason for the trauma.

Annually, in the United States, one out of every eleven workers in private industry experiences a work-related injury or illness during his working life (Garg, 1996). The Bureau of Labor statistics indicate that over fifty-five percent of these claims involve cumulative trauma injuries (Grant & Brisbin, 1992). It became apparent to employers that investment in ergonomic changes to the workstation was needed and would benefit their workers. By keeping workers healthy, production increases, which in turn increases profits and morale. This reduces employee turnover, resulting in more long-term skilled workers and lower new hiring and training costs.

## WORKSTATION PRINCIPLES

Many of today's jobs must be performed at a computer work area, often a "shared" workstation. Change, variation, and adjustment to fit the individual are basic to the well-being of the workers (Franchi & Fleck, 1994; Phair, 1995). Workstations should accommodate users of many different heights, weights, and individual needs. There are many areas to the average workstation, all of which need to be assessed individually. Both space and furniture must be designed to reduce employee fatigue and discomfort (Grant & Brisbin, 1992). Future technologies, such as voice recognition systems, and old technologies, such as the user's corrective lenses, should be addressed. The work area should be well lit, comfortable, and free of sounds.

The human is the most important component of any system because humans drive the process. So, the human must be accommodated first. It is important to verify the actual time the user spends in front of the computer. If the workstation is used frequently to constantly (thirty-three to one hundred percent of work time), this workstation, combined with the arrangement of items, may have a potential negative impact on staff. Cumulative trauma disorders (CTDs) have been associated with users who work for long periods of time at poorly constructed or poorly arranged workstations.

## RISK FACTORS

Marvin J. Dainoff, director of the Center for Ergonomic Research at Miami University, maintains that cumulative trauma disorders happen as the result of four risk factors, acting in combination (Franchi & Fleck, 1994):

1. High rates of repetition
2. Awkward posture
3. Use of excessive force
4. Lack of adequate rest and recovery

Many painful injuries are the result of improper posturing and mechanical stresses on the limbs, back, and legs. These usually begin with wrist complaints, associated with long-term use of keyboards in incorrect positions. Coupled with wrist pain, other symptoms such as normal fatigue, headaches, tingling in the upper extremities, and localized pain become more pronounced and more severe as time passes. Usually, the first signs of CTD are ignored, but as the symptoms progress and become more painful, the user surrenders to long-term physical therapy, medications to decrease the inflammation, a workers' compensation claim, and quite possibly another job or even another profession.

Ergonomically correct posture will assist in arranging work tasks and make the use of a computer or writing surface more efficient, with less stress to the entire body. Each workstation should be designed and analyzed by a person who is professionally trained in ergonomics, but with a basic assessment, users themselves can make improvements with some very simple measurements.

## ANATOMY AND PHYSIOLOGY

In order to use a writing surface or a keyboard and monitor, one must sit or stand. Most workstations are equipped with a chair or stool. A chair directly supports good posture (Grant & Brisbin, 1992). In the past, there has been the belief that "sitting with an upright trunk meant sitting healthily," which was based on the concept that the spinal column of the sitting person should be "erect" or "upright," similar to that of a person in a normal upright standing position. Allison (1992) states:

> The individual's specific seat height is determined by establishing that both feet are comfortably flat on the floor, with minimum pressure, the calf of the leg is perpendicular to the floor, the knees slightly higher than the hips to reduce excess curvature in the lower back. The front edge of the chair's seat should be tilted slightly down to avoid pressure behind

the knees. The employee should sit well back in the seat to support the lower lumbar region.

The anatomy of the spinal column consists of bones, muscles, and nerves. There are five major areas of the spine—the cervical or upper back, the thoracic or middle back, the lumbar region or lower back, and the sacral and coccyx—which combined make up the sitting portion. Each individual bone, the vertebra, rests upon a lower one, cushioned by the spinal membrane or disk that lies between each. Pressure on the spinal disks in the lumbar region is dependent upon trunk posture and support. When standing at ease, the forces in the lumbar spine can be measured at 330 newtons (N). This force increases by about 100 N when sitting on a stool without a backrest. There seems to be little difference in the measurement when someone is sitting erect with the arms hanging or sitting relaxed with the lower arms supported on the thighs. There is also an increase in pressure when sitting down versus standing, but the differences in posture are not very pronounced. The spinal forces are increased by typing (from 330 N up to 500 N), when the forearms and hands have to be lifted to keyboard height. The use of a lumbar backrest brings down the forces considerably. With only a five-centimeter backrest protrusion toward lumbar lordosis or tilting the hips and back at the waist slightly forward, the internal disk forces are cut in half (Grant & Brisbin, 1992).

## TASK, POSTURE, AND WORK ACTIVITIES

The successful ergonomic design of an office workstation depends on several interrelated parts. The task, the posture, and the work activities all interact. These three activities alone can be difficult to deal with, but these activities also must interact with existing furniture, equipment, and the environment. The combination of all these elements makes the picture more complicated.

## Reading

On a desk, material to be read is usually placed flat on the work surface, roughly at elbow height. If reading material needs to be reviewed more closely, it is usually lifted to a proper distance so the eyes can focus and it can be read easily. A ninety-degree-inclined surface has been recommended for easier reading (Kroemer, 1993). A document holder that uses a clip to hold papers or books and steadies the work is commonly used. A document holder is often placed too far to one side of the keyboard or writing surface, causing a constant twisted body posture and excessive lateral head and eye movement. Ideally, the document holder should be positioned as close to the middle of the user's work area as possible to reduce unnecessary head and eye movement. The disadvantage to using an upright document holder is that it may require more time when turning pages.

Research has shown that a user in a normal sitting posture prefers to look downward slightly, at angles between ten and forty degrees below the horizon, instead of looking straight ahead. When looking slightly downward, the head moves forward and the eyes settle downward, which appears to be the natural way the eyes focus with the least amount of effort. Conversely, the more one is forced to tilt the eyes upward, the more difficult it is to focus.

The top of the monitor should be at a level so that it is even with the user's forehead. At times it may be necessary to tilt the screen forward to reduce glare from overhead lighting. The recommended distance from the front edge of the work surface to the monitor screen is eighteen to twenty-five inches.

Eye fatigue can come from several causes. Indirect glare at a computer workstation is common. If a light source is reflected on the monitor's screen, this has the same effect as sunshine streaming in a window. The simplest remedy is to remove the light source, but if this is not possible, the screen may need to be repositioned, overhead lights dimmed by putting a louver over a ceiling light, a curtain pulled to shade a window, or task lighting repositioned to decrease glare. Asymmetric task lighting is available, either mounted to a base or with a clamp-on holder. Task lighting with a jointed arm makes it easy to position the light properly. To avoid creating a glare on the papers and keyboard, the bulb should be at least eighteen inches above the work surface.

The user might try avoiding white or light-colored clothing. All surrounding surfaces should have a flat, nonreflective finish (Phair, 1995). If these suggestions do not relieve the problem, there are filters that can be placed over the monitor screen that reduce the intensity of the light waves passing through the monitor, thus improving contrast. Other filters let light pass through only in certain directions, thus limiting access to only certain eye positions.

## Corrective Lenses

Eye fatigue also can be noted in users who wear corrective lenses to aid in reading the monitor. Using these lenses incorrectly can generate new problems. This is particularly true with "reading glasses." If the user has Presbyopia, assistive reading glasses are commonly prescribed. Magnification glasses can be purchased in most drug stores to help those who do not wear other prescriptive corrective lenses.

Reading glasses are very useful for a viewing distance of about forty to fifty centimeters or fifteen to nineteen inches and with a downward tilt of the eyes of approximately twenty-five degrees. Most computer monitors are further away and probably not in a downward position. In the attempt to focus, the user must squint or move the head closer to the correct focusing distance. Squinting leads to eye fatigue, and stretching the neck promotes muscle tension. These problems are even more pronounced if one wears bifocals or trifocals, where the lowest section of the glasses are meant for reading.

Because of the way these glasses are ground, the user is forced to tilt the head upward and back in order to get the display on the screen focused, potentially causing severe neck and shoulder muscular tension and headaches.

The solution is to wear full-sized corrective lens ground to the correct viewing distance for the workstation. Tell the optometrist that these glasses are to be used specifically for monitor viewing. Measure the distance from the user to the monitor screen before any changes are made in the corrective lenses. Inform the optometrist of this distance and the level of the monitor screen. While it may be costly for some workers to purchase another pair of glasses, it is much less costly than neck pain and headaches.

## Keyboards

Computer keyboard configuration was fashioned after the traditional typewriter keyboard. It is largely unchanged, except that today's computer keyboard may have over one hundred keys (Kroemer, 1993). The manual typewriter's keyboard was originally designed in an upright position, with rows of keys on different levels so that the type bars would not get tangled if struck in rapid sequence. The columns of keys run diagonally from left to right, which was also necessary on early typewriters due to the mechanical constraints on the type bars. The keys were arranged in straight sideways rows to accommodate the machine, but with little thought of the shape of the fingertips, which are not straight across. Today's keyboard must be operated with the hands pronated (thumbs down) due to the horizontal arrangement of the rows of keys.

Recommendations for keyboard improvements have been proposed by the industry. These include the relocation of some letters and the splitting of the keyboard into one half for the left hand and one half for the right hand, making the center section higher than the outsides. These changes would decrease fatigue to the fingers and hands, but there is a huge learning curve that must be taken into consideration for the typists.

In the computer workstation, the keyboard should be at a level so that the elbows are bent at seventy to ninety degrees (while arms are maintained at the sides of the body), with shoulders relaxed and wrists maintained in a straight (neutral) position. The use of wrist rests (four inches or wider) that extend beyond the wrist toward the forearm may be required for additional support and proper positioning.

## Chairs

The chair seat supports the weight of the entire upper body and should make the user feel comfortable and secure. The seatpan should be slightly concave to support the legs (Phair, 1995). Hard surfaces generate pressure points on the bony prominences of the skeleton, which can be avoided with upholstery, cushions, or other surfaces that can be adjusted to cushion body contours. The front edge of the chair seat should not put pressure on the back of the knees. The height of the seat must be widely adjustable, lowered to fifteen inches and raised to twenty-three inches to accommodate people with short and long lower legs. These adjustments should be easy to make while sitting in the chair.

When seated in a chair, the user's knees should be bent and level with his hips. Feet should be flat on the floor or resting comfortably on a footrest. The footrest must be adjustable for comfort. If feet are allowed to dangle, pressure is put on the back of the legs, cutting off circulation and causing numbness and tingling.

Backrests support some weight of the upper trunk, arms, and head, allowing muscles to relax. A backrest should be as large as the chair can accommodate. Recommendations of thirty-three inches high, and at least twelve inches wide, will fit chairs with a complete back. These backrests should provide support from the head and neck area down to the lumbar region of the back. A lumbar cushion/roll may be attached to the back of the chair to provide additional low back support. This modification may also be used to decrease the chair seat depth if necessary. A foam wedge can be placed on the chair seat to provide proper seat tilt and assist in proper knee/hip positioning. Halfback chairs may benefit from adjustments and a lumbar cushion/roll made to fit on these chairs.

When in proper alignment, the lower back should maintain contact with the back of the chair, with a seat width of about seventeen to nineteen inches. The low back support on the chair back (usually the bottom half) should be positioned in the low back (lumbar) curve. The lumbar support must be six to nine inches high and twelve to fourteen inches wide. The seat should tilt five to ten degrees toward the front, causing the lower back to move forward, relieving strain. Users with poor posture may feel uncomfortable with proper chair positioning and supports at first. Encourage them to try these new postures. The body's muscles must relearn the correct position. Once the users become accustomed to the supports, they will feel less tired by the end of the day.

## Armrests

Armrests should be available at the discretion of the user. Some users find that armrests hinder arm movement and get in the way when getting into and out of the chair. Armrests tend to strike work surfaces when users attempt to rotate the chair, while seated, in close proximity to the work surface. This can cause jarring of the back and lower back pain (Grant & Brisbin, 1992).

Sometimes short armrests, or no armrests at all, are preferable. If used, they should support the weight of hands, arms, and even portions of the upper trunk and head. They must be well located and suitable for load bearing.

Armrests on chairs can be up to twelve inches long and three inches wide. Make sure the arms of the chair can fit easily under the desk. Soft padding and smooth fabric protect the forearm and elbow areas from pressure points and harsh skin abrasions.

Adjustable armrests should move up and down about five inches. Armrests are only recommended for individuals who prefer to use them.

## Footrests

The user's feet should rest flat on the floor or on a footrest. Footrests or footstools are usually used if the chair cannot be adjusted correctly for the feet to be supported. The footrest should be large enough to allow the user to move his feet and change the posture of the legs under the work surface. A footrest or footstool should be portable and adjustable, approximately sixteen inches long, and a minimum of twelve inches wide. It should provide adequate support to the feet and legs, while being easy to adjust in two-inch increments (usually three- to six-inch adjustments).

## The Desk

The height of the desk must have the ability to be adjusted several inches. Allison (1992) recommends using only adjustable furniture. The surface height should range from twenty-three to thirty-two and one-half inches from the floor, depending on the size of the employee and the work being done.

## Extending and Reaching

To minimize overextending and overreaching, orient all frequently performed tasks within the "work zone." This zone is similar to that occupied by a desk blotter. With elbows maintained at the sides of the body, the front and side areas occupy this space. Frequently performed tasks should be oriented on the side of most use, which usually depends on hand dominance. Here are some examples to note:

- If the user is right-handed, the telephone, notepads, and pencils should be accessible from the right side of the desk. This helps to avoid extending and reaching across the body or bending and straining the head to one side.
- The habit of holding the telephone receiver with the neck and shoulder (no hands) should be discouraged. Shoulder cradles assist some, but still the neck and shoulder muscles can be strained, as they are being pulled to one side.
- The wastepaper basket should be in a position of easy access. Twisting, bending, and reaching should be avoided with this repetitious movement.
- If a light pen is used for computer screen selections, it is helpful to have an armrest or handrest adjacent and anterior to the screen, but it should not interfere with the user's visual field (MacArthur & Sampson, 1985).

- If the monitor uses a mouse for screen selection, locate the mouse on the dominant side of the user. Mouse pads and supports are helpful in keeping the wrist and forearm in a neutral position.
- Something as simple as where the user places his coffee cup may be of importance. Twisting and reaching repeatedly should be avoided.
- Be aware of overhead shelves and the overextending of the shoulders and arms. Avoid having to pull or lift heavy books or manuals from a shelf overhead. Use two hands to support heavy objects to avoid overuse of the wrist and lower arm.
- Keep needed materials within the waist to shoulder level. When reaching for an object, address it straight on, not at angle reaching over and around other objects.

## Printers

Printers need to be either close enough to readily gather documents easily without twisting and overextension, or they should be far enough away to ensure that the user must get up and walk to gather documents. The noise of the printer must be considered in the user's environment (MacArthur & Sampson, 1985). Printer covers are available to dampen noise with older printers.

Other noises, such as cooling fans or transformers, also need to be assessed. All the sound levels combined should be kept at or below sixty decibels, if possible, in the work space (Kroemer, 1993).

## CHANGING THE WORKPLACE IS NOT ENOUGH

Poor workplace design is often the major source for CTDs. Ergonomic design of work tasks can reduce or remove some of the risks, but the workplace may not be the cause of the employee's problem. Poor employee posture habits and body mechanics frequently cause CTD. The addition of ergonomic furniture and assistive devices will not help if the employee will not use them properly. Osterman (1996) suggests some other solutions:

- Information and training about body positions that eliminate the opportunity for repetitive stress injuries to occur can be made available.
- Job task rotation costs very little and can be extremely effective, according to some experts. Workers simply swap jobs occasionally during the workday to vary the physical demands.
- Frequent switching between standing and sitting positions is another form of task rotation, reducing the net stress to any specific muscle or skeletal group.
- Another low-cost option is routine stretching. These types of exercises must meet certain prerequisites to be safe and effective, but they have proven to be successful

for many employees and employers. Best of all, evidence shows these exercises do not reduce worker productivity.

• Basic personal fitness is another factor employers should take into account. Maximum ergonomic benefits can occur only when there is a joint partnership between employer and employee to maintain a healthy body, a productive work environment, and a positive attitude.

• Lastly, Osterman (1996) says, "I tell people to lighten up on their intensity all the way around. This helps the workers who hold their pencils too tight or furiously pound on computer keyboards."

## STRETCHES

The advancement of telecommunications and computer technology allows people to have the information they need at their fingertips, literally. Unfortunately, spending prolonged periods of time working at a computer or in any one position can affect the entire body. Adopting a stretching program on a frequent basis, once every hour is recommended, will enhance flexibility and circulation, and reduce fatigue of all muscle groups. These stretches should be done several times per day. Pay close attention to your breathing. You cannot hold your breath and relax at the same time.

### Neck

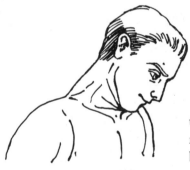

**Chin to Chest.** Gently lower the head so the chin touches the chest. Feel the pull in the back of the neck. Hold here for 20 seconds. Do not forget to breathe. Do this 3 times.

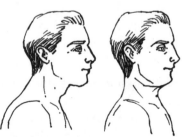

**Chin Tuck.** With head erect, pull the chin back toward the shoulders. Feel the pull in the top of the shoulders. Hold for 5 seconds. Repeat 5 times.

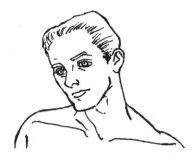

**Ear to Shoulder.** Very gently, with head erect, lower your head to the side and down to the shoulder, as if to touch the ear to the shoulder. Keep the shoulders level. Feel the stretch in the opposite side of the neck. Hold for 20 seconds. Move to the other side and stretch the ear toward the shoulder. Hold for 20 seconds.

## Shoulder

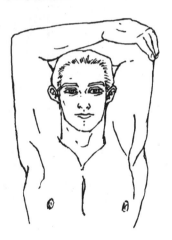

**Shoulder Pull.** Place both arms over the head and, bending at elbow, grab the opposite arm at the elbow. Gently pull the opposite arm. The arms will be behind the head. Head and shoulders should be level and in a neutral position. Hold the stretch for 20 seconds. Move to the opposite arm. Again, gently pull for 20 seconds. Repeat this 3 more times. Feel the stretch in the upper arm and shoulder.

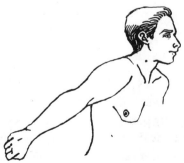

**Reach Behind.** Sitting or standing, gently reach the arm behind the back to a comfortable stretch. Feel the stretch in the shoulder, arm, and neck areas. Move to the opposite arm. Repeat this 3 times, holding the stretch for 20 seconds.

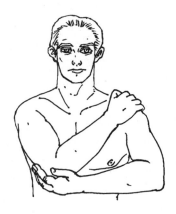

**Arm Across Chest.** Sitting or standing, place the right hand on the left shoulder. With the left hand, gently stretch the right shoulder and upper arm. Hold for 20 seconds. Move to the opposite arm. Repeat this 3 times.

## Forearm

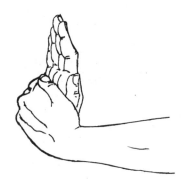

**Wrist Extension.** With arm out in front of the body, lift wrist up. Using the other hand, gently apply pressure on the palm of the hand, pulling it toward the body. Hold for 5 seconds. Feel the stretch in the forearm. Repeat with the other arm.

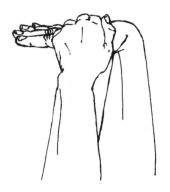

**Wrist Flexion.** With arms out in front of the body, let the wrists drop downward. Using one hand to pull the opposite hand, gently put pressure on the back of the hand toward the body. Feel the stretch in the top of the arm. Hold for 5 seconds. Repeat 3 more times.

# Hand

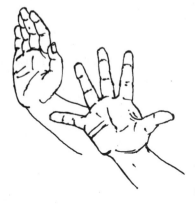

**Finger Spread.** Hold each hand out in front of the body. Spread fingers as wide as possible. Hold for 5 seconds. Repeat 3 more times.

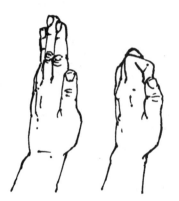

**Finger Fold.** Hold each hand out in front of the body. Curl fingers inward, making them clawlike. Hold for 5 seconds. Repeat 3 more times.

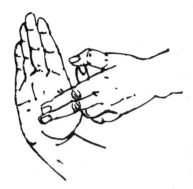

**Thumb Push.** Hold hand out in front of the body, flexing at the wrist. Using your other hand, put gentle pressure on the thumb area, stretching out the thumb from the fingers. Hold for 5 seconds. Repeat 3 more times.

By implementing the recommendations discussed in this chapter, the time one spends at a workstation and performing work tasks may be dramatically enhanced while preventing potential problems with cumulative trauma disorders.

# REFERENCES

Allison, G. (1992). Of ergonomics and office furniture. *The Office, 1992*(6), 12–14.

Anchin, J. S. (1996). Small business insurance: What you need to know. *Westchester County Business Journal, 35*(16), 37.

Franchi, K., & Fleck, R. A. (1994) Ergonomic improvements in the office environment. *Business Horizons, 37*(2), 75–84.

Garg, A. (1995). *Industrial safety. Microsoft Encarta 96 Encyclopedia.* Funk & Wagnalls Corporation.

Grant, C. B., & Brisbin, R. E. (1992). *Workplace wellness.* New York: Van Norstrand Reinhold.

Kroemer, K. H. E. (1993). Fitting the workplace to the human and not vice versa. *Industrial Engineering, 25*(3), 56–61.

MacArthur, A. M., & Sampson, M. R. (1985). Screen design of a hospital information system. *Nursing Clinics of North America, 20*(3), 471–486.

Osterman, N. (1996). Performance of mobile worker tied to flexible office design. *Supervision, 57*(6), 12–15.

Phair, M. (1995). Computer ease: Guidelines for setting up a comfortable workstation at home. *Home Mechanix, 91*(800), 39–44.

Rademaker, K. (1992). The "bandage brigade" no more: Occupational health nursing. *Occupational Hazards, 54*(4), 51–55.

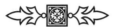

# APPENDIX

# Acronyms

| | |
|---|---|
| ADT | Admission-discharge-transfer |
| AHA | American Hospital Association |
| ANA | American Nurses Association |
| ANSI | American National Standards Institute |
| ASCII | American Standard Code of Information Interchange |
| BASIC | Beginners All-Purpose Symbolic Instruction Code |
| BBS | Bulletin board system |
| Bit | Binary digit |
| CAD | Computer-aided design |
| CD | Compact disk |
| CEO | Chief executive officer |
| CHIM | Council on Hospital Information Management |
| CHMIS | Community Health Management Information System |
| CHIN | Comunity health information network |
| CIO | Chief information officer |

| COBOL | Common Business-Oriented Language |
|---|---|
| COLD | Computer output to laser disk |
| CORBA | Common object request broker architecture |
| CPR | Computer-based patient record |
| CPRI | Computer-based Patient Record Institute |
| CPT-4 | Current procedural terminology |
| CPU | Central processing unit |
| CRT | Cathode-ray tube |
| CTD | Cumulative trauma disorder |
| DB | Database |
| DBMS | Database management systems |
| DOS | Disk operating system |
| DRG | Diagnostic-related group |
| DSU | Digital service unit |
| EDI | Electronic data interchange (standardizing data exchange) |
| EDIFACT | Electronic Data Interchange for Administration, Commerce and Transport |
| EDS | Executive decision system |
| EFT | Electronic funds transfer |
| EIS | Executive information system |
| E-mail | Electronic mail |
| EMS | Emergency medical services |
| EPROM | Erasable programmable read-only memory |
| FORTRAN | Formula translation |
| FTE | Full-time employee |
| FTP | File transfer protocol |
| GUI | Graphical user interface |
| HCFA | Health Care Financing Administration |
| HEDIS | Health Plan Employer Data and Information Set |
| HIMSS | Hospital Information Management System Society |
| HIS | Health information systems |
| HISPP | Health Care Informatics Standards Planning Panel |
| HL7 | Health Level Seven |
| HMO | Health maintenance organization |
| HTML | Hypertext markup language |
| http | Hypertext transfer protocol |
| IBM | International Business Machines |
| ICD-9-CM | International Classification of Diseases, 9th revision, Clinical Modification |
| IDS | Integrated delivery system |

| | |
|---|---|
| IM | Information management |
| INS | Informatics nursing specialist |
| I/O | Input/output |
| IP | Internet protocol |
| IRDS | Information resource dictionary systems |
| ISDN | Integrated services digital network |
| ISO | International Standards Organization |
| IT | Information technology |
| JCAHO | Joint Commission on Accreditation of Healthcare Organizations |
| LAN | Local area network |
| MIME | Multipurpose Internet mail extension |
| MIPS | Millions of instructions per second |
| MIS | Management information system |
| MPI | Master patient index |
| MSO | Management services organization |
| NMDS | Nursing minimum data set |
| OCR | Optical character recognition |
| OLE | Object linking and embedding |
| OS | Operating system |
| PACS | Picture archiving and communications system |
| PC | Personal computer |
| POC | Point of care |
| POS | Professional operating system (DEC product) |
| PPO | Physician provider organization |
| PROM | Programmable read-only memory |
| RAID | Redundant array of inexpensive disk |
| RAM | Random access memory |
| RAS | Reliability, availability, serviceability |
| RBRVS | Resource-based relative value studies |
| RFI | Request for information |
| RFP | Request for proposal |
| ROM | Read-only memory |
| SMDS | Switched network management protocol |
| SNA | Systems network architecture |
| SNMP | Simple network management protocol |
| Snomed | Systematized Nomenclature of Human and Veterinary Medicine |
| SQL | Standard query language |
| TCP | Transmission control protocol |
| UCDS | Uniform Clinical Data Set (used for Medicare Peer Review process) |
| VAN | Value-added network |

| | |
|---|---|
| VDU | Visual display unit |
| WAIS | Wide area information server |
| WAN | Wide area network |
| WEDI | Work Group for Electronic Data Interchange (cochaired by Blue Cross/Blue Shield Association) |
| WHO | World Health Organization |

# APPENDIX

# Glossary

**Access network**   The connection of a small remote site to the backbone so that remote users can fully participate in network computing.

**Admission-discharge-transfer (ADT) system**   A software program used to keep track of patients from time of admission until they are discharged.

**Alpha site**   A location where hardware or software products are initially tested. This usually serves as a laboratory environment. The next step is beta testing before the products are released for commercial distribution.

**Application program**   A computer program written to solve a specific problem or to perform a specific task.

**Application server**   A special type of file server optimized for a specific task, such as communications or database management, that uses higher-end hardware than a typical file server.

**Archie**   An abbreviation for archive, it is a protocol for searching at any site on the Internet that may be accessed through a file transfer protocol (FTP). Using Archie,

187

you know what is available at each FTP site, and it lets you search for files about particular subjects.

**Artificial intelligence**   Developing and applying computers that perform in ways comparable to humans, emphasizing symbolic rather than numeric reasoning and thus emulating human problem solving.

**Asynchronous transfer mode**   An ultrahigh-speed switching technology that simultaneously can route voice, data, and video communications over fiber-optic and other telecommunication lines at rates that eventually reach billions of bits per second.

**Attachment**   Additional documentation required by a payer as an addendum to either a paper or electronic claim as a condition of payment.

**Audit trail**   A security component of an operating system that constantly maintains a log of which system users accessed which files at which times. If a file is feared compromised, a system operator can consult the individual file's audit trail to determine who accessed the file in question.

**Backbone**   The part of a network that links several work groups of local area networks together in one building or links together the local area networks of several buildings on one campus.

**Backbone network**   A number of multiport routers connected to each other by LAN or WAN connections. A router backbone serves as the main information conduit for major sites in an enterprise and usually does so at very high speed with high volumes of traffic.

**Backup**   A duplicate copy of a file or program. Backups of material are made on disk or cassette in case something happens to the original.

**Bandwidth**   A measurement of transmission capacity. The greater the bandwidth, the greater the information-carrying capability of the transmission medium. Analog transmission is measured in cycles per second. Digital transmission is measured in bits of information per second.

**Batch EDI**   A one-direction transmission of grouped data. Usually the only immediate response from the receiver is verification that the transmission has been received or that a problem has occurred. The originator receives a response later through a separate transmission. Batch EDI is a more basic approach than on-line, interactive EDI.

**Batch processing**   A mode of processing in which any program submitted to the computer is either run to completion or aborted. No interactive communication between program and user is possible.

**Baud**   Unit of measurement of transmission speed, equivalent to bits per second in serial transmission. Used by microcomputer.

**Beginner's All-Purpose Symbolic Instruction Code (BASIC)**   A popular computer language invented at Dartmouth for educational purposes. An easy-to-learn, easy-to-use language.

**Beta site**   A location where real-world field testing is performed before a hardware or software product is formally released for commercial distribution.

**Binary number system**   Number system made up of the digits 0 and 1, "the language of the computer."

**Bisynchronous communications**   A protocol used extensively in mainframe computer networks. Both the sending and receiving devices must be synchronized before data transmission begins. Data is collected into a package known as a frame; each frame contains leading and trailing characters that allow the computers to synchronize their clocks.

**Bit**   <u>Bi</u>nary di<u>git</u> (0 or 1).

**Bookmark**   Most Web browsers allow users to create bookmarks for interesting Web pages. Users can then revisit these pages directly, without traversing multiple links, by choosing the bookmarks from a menu in the Web browser.

**Bridge**   A simple, limited function device for connecting a series of two or more segments of a local area network. A bridge has a physical interface or port for each LAN to which it is connected. Bridges are a relatively inefficient means of interconnecting LANs, but they are necessary for some unroutable protocols.

**Broadband network**   A network capable of transporting voice, interactive full-motion video, and data services. Technically, the network must be able to transmit 1.5 million or more bits of information per second.

**Browser**   Client software that enables users to navigate between host computers connected to a network to request and display data. Such software is free or inexpensive and can be downloaded from the Internet or obtained from a company that provides access to the Internet. Common browsers are Netscape's Navigator and Microsoft's Internet Explorer.

**Bug**   An error in a program or an equipment fault.

**Bulletin board**   Informal information exchanges that allow a user to post a message that can be read by a large group of members. The reader has an opportunity to write back responses.

**Bulletin board system (BBS)**   A computerized dial-in meeting and announcement system that allows people to participate in discussions, upload and download files, and make announcements, without requiring the use of concurrent connections to the computer.

**Bus topology**   A configuration that allows all nodes on a network to receive the same message through the network at the same time.

**Byte**   Eight bits make up a byte (a letter, symbol, or number).

**Cathode-ray tube (CRT)**   A tube in a television set or video display monitor.

**Cell**   A packet of information that is fixed in size, containing a header that holds path information used to relay it through switching devices or networks.

**Central processing unit (CPU)**   Internal part of the computer that contains the circuits that control and perform the execution of instructions. It is made up of memory, arithmetic/logic unit, and control unit.

**Chip**   An integrated circuit made by etching a myriad of transistors and other electronic components onto a wafer of silicon a fraction of an inch on a side.

**Classification**   A systematic arrangement of classes; a structural framework arranged according to similar groups.

**Classification system**   An arrangement of the elements of a subject into groups according to preestablished criteria. For example, in ICD-9-CM, the diseases are arranged in chapters, sections, categories, and subcategories for tabulating events or episodes of morbidity and mortality.

**Client**   The system (software application running on a piece of hardware) that initiates the process or requests services in a client-server computing arrangement.

**Client-server**   A style of distributed computing that allows several local area network-based PCs or workstations, known as clients, to share access to a more powerful server computer. With this approach, processes are divided between two systems that work together to perform a task, such as getting information from a database.

**Clinical decision support**   The capability of a system to provide key data to physicians and other clinicians in response to certain rule-based triggers.

**Clinical information system**   An information system that collects, stores, and/or transmits information that is used to support clinical applications. Billing systems and other financial systems would not be considered clinical information systems.

**Coaxial cable**   A transmission line with a central core that conducts electricity. This core is surrounded by insulation, followed by another layer of conducting material. Coaxial cable, which is used in the cable TV industry, can transmit more information than a pair of twisted copper wires, commonly used for telephone communication.

**Coding system**   A structured set of characters used to represent data items.

**Common object request broker architecture (CORBA)**   A type of object-oriented network and applications standard for networked "object stores." CORBA allows heterogeneous data and applications to be encapsulated within an "object" to provide a common framework for sharing among other CORBA-compliant applications.

**Community health information network (CHIN)**   An organization that offers electronic connections that enable all providers, payers, and purchasers of care to exchange financial, clinical, and administrative information in a defined geographic region.

**Compiler**   A translation program that converts high-level instructions into a set of binary instructions (object code) for direct processor execution. Any high-level program requires a compiler or an interpreter.

**Computer**   An electronic device capable of taking in, putting out, storing internally, and processing data under the control of changeable processing instructions within the device.

**Computer-based patient record (CPR)**   All of the data and images collected over the course of a patient's health history.

**Computer-based patient record system**   A computerized system that captures, stores, retrieves, and transmits patient-specific health care–related data, including clinical, administrative, and payment data.

**Computer literacy**   A term used to indicate knowledge of what a computer can do, how it works, how it is used to solve problems, and the limitations of the computer.

**Computer output to laser disk (COLD)**   A document imaging application that takes electronic data directly from information systems and stores it along with document images. COLD systems use form overlay functions to make electronic data appear like a document and allow the printing of data, so it looks like a paper version of the appropriate document.

**Control key**   A key that executes commands, in conjunction with other keys pressed simultaneously.

**Control unit**   The internal part of a computer (found in the CPU) that monitors the sequence of operations for all parts of the computer.

**Cooperative processing**   Another term for client-server computing that is used in association with systems or hardware made by IBM Corporation.

**Current processing**   Another term for client-server computing that is used in association with systems or hardware made by IBM Corporation.

**Cursor**   A patch of light or other visual indicator on a screen that shows you where you are in the text.

**Data**   Recorded facts on which arithmetic and logical processes are performed.

**Database (DB)**   An organized collection of data or information; interrelated files with records organized and stored together in a computer system.

**Database server**   A computer that stores data centrally for network users. It often uses client-server software to distribute the processing of data among itself and other workstations on the network.

**Data dictionary**   A description of all the data fields with an information system, for example, name of patient, name of test, test results.

**Data element**   The smallest unit of data that has meaning without interpretation; a raw fact, material, or observation. For example, patient's name, date of birth, and so on.

**Data entry**   The act of entering information in a computer by keyboard, optical scanning, or voice recognition.

**Data mining**   A technique that uncovers new information from existing information by probing mammoth data sets.

**Data repository**   In a health care setting, a database that brings together information from various venues of patient information available where and when it is needed, such as, from multiple sites within an integrated delivery system. A repository stores on-line transaction information and serves as a warehouse for research efforts.

**Data set**   Defined sets of information collected for a specific purpose; a directory. For example, a uniform bill data set of information collected for the purpose of claims processing.

**Digital**   A computer that uses numbers to solve problems by performing arithmetic and logical processes on data.

**Digital dictation**   A system that stores digitized voice files on a computer's hard drive, allowing them to be easily accessed and managed by transcriptionists. Often, verbal prompts are employed to guide the user through the system. Because the recording is computer-based, transcriptionists can slow down the replay of the file without distortion, which occurs when a tape is played at a slower speed.

**Digital service unit (DSU)**   A device used in digital transmission for connecting data terminal equipment, such as a router, to a network. DSUs often are coupled with channel service units that allocate channels from a high-speed data circuit.

**Digital transmission**   Converts sound waves and other information into binary computer code, which is a series of zeroes and ones. The information is sent in digital format, then it is converted back to its original format when it reaches its destination. This provides sharper, clearer, and faster transmission than analog transmission, because it can be repeated without introducing noise.

**Directory services**   A health care telecommunications network value-added feature that helps expedite the delivery of a transaction to the intended destination. The network will look up the destination address by multiple identifiers and route the transaction or return to the requester the routing information.

**Disease management**   The prospective development of interventions designed for patients with particular conditions. Health measures are designed to alter the course of the condition to both prevent exacerbation of the illness and improve the patient's quality of life. Research for disease management purposes requires clinical data stored in computer databases.

**Disk**   An external storage medium that is a flat, circular magnetic surface used to store data. The data is represented by the presence or absence of magnetized spots.

**Disk drive**   The device used to access or store information via a disk.

**Diskless workstation**   A networked computer that does not have any local disk storage capability. The computer boots and loads all its programs from the network file server. Diskless workstations are particularly valuable when sensitive information is processed because information cannot be copied from the file server onto a local disk.

**Distributed computing**   A style of computing in which computing resources are spread throughout the organization, distributing data and processing chores to PCs, workstations, minicomputers, and mainframes throughout an enterprise. Client-server systems typically are distributed computing, but distributed computing need not involve client-server systems. One use of distributed computing is in a distributed database, which allows information stored on separate systems to be accessed by disparate members of a network, creating a virtual central repository.

**Documentation**   Refers to the orderly presentation, organization, and communication of recorded specialized knowledge in order to maintain a complete record of reasons for changes in variables. Documentation is necessary, not so much to give maximum utility, as to give an unquestionable historical reference record.

**Document imaging**   The use of scanners to digitize paper documents and their information so the data can be stored on computer systems.

**Download**   The process of transferring information stored in a remote computer to a local computer.

**Dumb terminal**   A computing unit that has a keyboard and screen but no internal memory or processor; it functions as an input/display unit only. It can function only because it is attached to another unit, typically a mainframe computer, that serves as the processor.

**Duplexing**   The process of operating identical disk drives or servers to maintain a fault-tolerant network environment. If the primary system fails, the secondary system automatically takes over, thus ensuring continued and uninterrupted network operations.

**Electronic Data Interchange for Administration, Commerce and Transport (EDI-FACT)**   United Nations rules that comprise a set of internationally agreed upon standards, directories, and guidelines for computer-to-computer exchange (either real-time or batch) via a standard on-line transmission method.

**Electronic data interchange (EDI)**   An exchange of data in electronic form, usually point-to-point, across a telephone line.

**Electronic funds transfer (EFT)**   The paperless exchange of money through electronic data interchange. This exchange is enabled through the use of the American National Standards Institute's ASC X12 835 standard format.

**Electronic mail (E-mail)**   The use of a network to transmit text messages, memos, graphics, and reports. Messages can be sent to one or more persons, a defined group, or all users on a system.

**Eligibility**   The determination of whether a payer will cover a person's treatment. The answer may depend on who the provider is or the type of services suggested.

**Encoder**   An automated coding system that takes codes entered by coding staff and, using a series of built-in prompts, enables them to code more accurately and specifically. Prompts perform such tasks as resequencing codes by priority, verifying the relationship between grouped codes, and suggesting additional related codes not initially entered by coding staff.

**Encryption**   A data security approach that changes readable text into a vast series of characters and numbers using complex mathematical algorithms. Computers on either end of a encrypted message have "keys" that decrypt data into its original format.

**End station**   A computer connected to a network. Network end stations include PCs, workstations, minicomputers, and mainframe computers.

**Enterprisewide network**   A network that connects every computer in every location of an organization and runs the enterprise's mission-critical application. Many integrated health care delivery systems are building enterprisewide networks to tie together multiple delivery sites.

**Ethernet**   A network protocol and cabling scheme with a transfer rate of 10 megabits per second. It uses a bus topology capable of connecting, as many as 1,024 PCs and workstations within each main branch. Network nodes are connected by coaxial cable, fiber-optic cable, or twisted-pair wiring.

**Executive information system (EIS)**   A software program that draws together information from various segments of an organization's operations to help administrators better manage the organization.

**Expert system**   A program that uses a set of rules to construct a reasoning process. An expert system, sometimes called a rules-based system, can reach conclusions and generate new data. In other words, it can learn.

**Fast packet**   A data transmission format through which blocks of data are sent over a network. With this method, called packet switching, these blocks of information are quickly and simultaneously routed and transmitted from many different network users over lines, cables, or some other medium.

**Fiber-distributed data interface**   A specification that allows transmission on fiber-optic networks of as much as 100 megabits per second over a dual-token ring topology. That speed is close to the internal speed of most computers, which makes it a good choice to serve as a super backbone linking two or more local area networks. FDDI is suited to systems that require the transfer of large amounts of information, such as medical images.

**Fiber-optic technology**   A communications approach that uses light pulses traveling through hair-thin glass strands to transmit information. This provides higher-quality transmission and greater capacity than traditional copper wire.

**File server**   A minicomputer that functions as a traffic director as various users communicate with each other, request access to files on the shared disk, and use shared peripherals such as printers. It manages the network.

**File transfer protocol (FTP)**   A standard, high-level protocol under the transmission control protocol/Internet protocol (TCP/IP) suite used to control the exchange of files between two hosts or from one computer to another.

**Firewall**   A hardware and software combination that is used to prevent outsiders from tampering with the internal computer system of an Internet user. The firewall acts as a gateway, monitoring traffic between an Internet site and the Internet, ferreting out and blocking unauthorized access.

**Firmware**   Computer instructions that are located in read-only memory (ROM). These instructions can be accessed but not altered.

**Floppy disk**   A flexible plastic disk enclosed in a protective envelope used to store information.

**Format**   The structured arrangement of data fields and elements that constitute a particular transaction or the organization of data in such as way as to have a specific, agreed-upon meaning among users of the data. Proprietary formats are privately owned and used and agreed on by individual users, whereas standard formats are uniform to an entire industry.

**Frame**   A unit of data that varies widely in size. It contains a packet, plus fields containing information for checking errors and performing other functions.

**Frame relay**   A high-speed packet switching service for moving blocks of data over a network. It can move large amounts of data quickly, operating at 56,000 to 1.5 million bits per second for such applications as imaging, file transfer, and data network interconnection.

**Friendly**   How easy a program or computer is to work with. A "user-friendly" program is one that takes little time to learn, that offers on-screen prompts, or that protects the user from making disastrous mistakes.

**Fuzzy logic**   A rules-based system that mimics human thought, enabling a computer to "think" in exact terms, rather than in a definitive, "either/or" manner. Fuzzy logic is a powerful way to combine traditional computing methods with symbolic reasoning.

**Gateway**   A shared connection between a local area network and a larger system, such as a mainframe computer or a large packet switching network, whose communication protocols are different. Usually slower than a bridge or router, a gateway is a combination of hardware and software with its own processor and memory used to perform protocol conversions.

**Genetic algorithm**   A program based on the rule of "survival of the fittest." A genetic algorithm examines data and determines by programmed stipulations which data best match a stated goal and which data do not. For example, a genetic algorithm can be used to judge which automated clinical protocols best match a provider's predefined clinical objectives.

**Gigabyte (GB)**   In computing, 1 billion bytes, or 1,000 megabytes. Gigabytes are used to represent large hard disk capacities.

**Gopher** An Internet browsing service in which information is organized by menus. It is also a protocol for the menu-based system of accessing documents on the Internet, or any program that implements this protocol.

**Graphical user interface (GUI)** A key component of client systems, the GUI is the set of menus, windows, control buttons, and other standard screen devices that are intended to make using a computer as intuitive as possible.

**Groupers** An automated coding system that classifies numeric codes representing diagnoses under appropriate diagnostic-related groups (DRGS). Groupers are crucial to successful coding and reimbursement, because they determine which types of complicating diagnoses and/or additional procedures affect a principal diagnosis and, based on that review, place the coded diagnosis or procedure into the appropriate DRG.

**Hard copy** Computer output printed on paper.

**HCFA Common Procedural Coding System (HCPCS)** A list of services, procedures, and supplies offered by physicians and other providers. HCPCS includes current procedural terminology codes, national alphanumeric codes, and local alphanumeric codes. Providers must use HCPCS to get paid by Medicare.

**HCFA 1500** A universal form, developed by the Health Care Financing Administration, that providers of services use to bill professional fees to health carriers. It is also known as the Uniform Health Insurance claim form. By law, it must be used for claims submitted to the Medicare program by individual health care practitioners.

**Head** The part of a magnetic storage unit (disk drive) that reads and writes information on the magnetic media.

**Health care informatics** A discipline that combines health care sciences and computer science.

**Health information infrastructure** An interconnected communications network consisting of a computer-based patient record system, a computerized knowledge based patient record systems, computerized knowledge based systems, and reference databases, all of which are connected through high-speed communications links using common definitions, codes, and forms.

**Health information systems (HIS)** A term used to describe overall hospital use of computers. For example, nursing systems, medical records, patient admittance and discharge, patient bed control, and so on.

**Health Level Seven (HL7)** A group establishing standards for the electronic exchange of text messages, including data on admissions, discharges, transfers, financial transactions, scheduling, and nursing management within health care provider organizations.

**Health Plan Employer Data and Information Set (HEDIS)** A core set of performance measures to assist employers and other health purchasers in understanding the value of health plan performance. HEDIS was developed by the National Committee for Quality Assurance.

**High-level languages**   Programming languages that are as close to writing English statements as possible.

**Home page**   On the World Wide Web, a display that usually identifies and describes the page owner and contains buttons with links to other pages. Using a mouse, a user can click on a button to go to an associated page. A home page is like a hypertext table of contents.

**Host**   Any computer on a network that is a repository for services to other computers on the network. It is common to have one host machine provide several services such as Web pages and Usenet group.

**Hub**   A hardware devise with many ports to which computers and peripheral devices are attached. There are three types of hubs: modular hubs, which have a chassis with several slots for various types of computer cards; stand-alone hubs, which contain a fixed number of ports; and stackable hubs, which allow several to be connected to serve as a single unit.

**Hypermedia**   Hypertext that includes some combination of pictures, sound, graphics, and moving images.

**Hypertext**   Documents on the World Wide Web and author-defined features called links or hotspots. Each of these, when selected by a user, connects the text to related items that may be located anywhere on the Internet.

**Hypertext markup language (HTML)**   The language that underpins the Web. It consists of a set of codes that can be added to plain text documents to indicate embedded images, links, hierarchical heading relationships, and more. HTML documents are interpreted by Web browsers and presented to end users as multimedia documents with hyperlinks. HTML also allows for the creation of forms and other enhancements to the basic document structure.

**Hypertext transfer protocol (http)**   A prefix to an Internet address that indicates to a Web browser that an HTML page is located at that address.

**Information resource dictionary systems (IRDS)**   A software tool that can be used to control, describe, protect, and access an organization's information resources. The IRDS is usually built through the combination of an organization's multiple data dictionaries.

**Input**   The data to be processed by the computer.

**Input/output (I/O)**   An input device such as a keyboard feeds information into the computer. Other input devices include voice input and light pen. An output device such as a printer or monitor takes information from the computer and turns it into a usable form. Modems, cassettes, and disks work in both directions, so they are I/O devices.

**Integrated delivery system (IDS)**   A group of affiliated provider sites, often with a single owner, that offers a continuum of care to those enrolled in managed care plans. These systems typically include hospitals, physicians, ambulatory care sites, and other care delivery venues.

**Integrated services digital network (ISDN)**   High-speed transmission technology that provides two 64,000-bits-per-second channels and a third lower-speed channel that can handle voice and data transmission simultaneously.

**Intelligent character recognition**   An advanced imaging technology that uses a scanning device to convert a wide variety of paper documents to electronic images that can be stored and manipulated on a computer.

**Intelligent hubs**   Hubs in which each port can be configured, monitored, or disabled without direct contact, for example, from a management console. They also allow network managers to gather information on operations, such as how many packets are passing through hubs and their individual ports.

**Interactive EDI**   Transactions that involve two-way, instantaneous communication. An interactive transaction is similar to a conversation; it is characterized by a requester logging into another computer system and receiving one or more responses while still on-line with that system.

**Interface**   An electronic connection between software programs operating on the same computer system or between two information systems. The term is also used to describe a software program that establishes or allows communication between otherwise incompatible programs or systems.

**Interface engine**   Software that permits the flow of information from one application to another within an organization without the need to develop point-to-point interfaces. The technology provides for the real-time translation, routing, and switching of data.

**Internal memory**   The internal storage of the computer, which is made up of ROM and RAM.

**International Classification of Diseases, 9th revision, Clinical Modification (ICD-9-CM)**   Codes used to classify patient treatment at hospitals. Medicare requires use of the code for providers who bill for both inpatient and ambulatory care, as well as itemized billing statements. The codes also are used to place patients into diagnostic-related groups. ICD-9-CM, published by the federal government, is a clinical modification of a World Health Organization compendium that serves as a standard for disease and procedure codes.

**International Standards Organization (ISO)**   An organization that sets computer and communications standards worldwide. It is best known for its Open Systems Interconnect reference model, which specifies how different computing devices can share data on a network. The model does this by defining seven layers, each delineating a subset of all local area network services.

**Internet**   The world's largest computer network of networks. The Internet uses transmission control protocol/Internet protocol (TCP/IP) to link government, university, and commercial institutions.

**Internet protocol (IP)**   The underlying transport protocol for the Internet suite of products. The Internet protocol is supported by an international user/developer community and has been developed with open standards. The entire suite is called the transmission control protocol/Internet protocol (TCP/IP), because the transmission control protocol and the Internet protocol are the two most fundamental protocols.

**Interoperability**   The ability to run application programs from different vendors across local, wide, and metropolitan area networks, giving users access to data and applications across heterogeneous networks. A network user need not know anything about the operating system or the configuration of the network hardware to gain access to data from the file server.

**Intranet**   Private computer networks that use Internet protocols and Internet-derived technologies, including World Wide Web browsers, Web servers, and Web languages to facilitate collaborative data sharing within an enterprise.

**Java**   A new programming language invented by Sun Microsystems Computer Company that is designed for writing programs that can be securely downloaded to a computer via the Internet and immediately run by a computer user. Using applets, tiny Java programs, Web pages can include functions such as calculators and audio or video samples.

**Jughead**   A tool used to search a specific gopher site.

**Jukebox**   A high-capacity storage device that uses an autochanger mechanism to mount or dismount optical disks.

**Kilobyte (KB)**   A term used to express 1,000. In the computer context, 16K = 16,000 bytes.

**Knowledge-based system**   A computer system that combines access to data and systematic use of logic rules and probabilistic statements that can help caregivers make better clinical decisions, for example, recognize out-of-range laboratory values or dangerous trends, associate symptoms with the correct diagnosis, select the optimal treatment approach.

**Language**   In computing and communications, a set of characters (symbols, alphabets, codes, and syntax), conventions, and rules used to convey ideas and information.

**Leased line**   A private communications channel leased from a common communications carrier. Leased lines are commonly used to connect distant terminals or printers to a central processing unit at another location or to a communications network.

**Legacy systems**   Computer applications that have been "inherited" through previous information system acquisitions and installations. Legacy systems run business applications that generally are not integrated with each other and are commonly monolith in design. The concepts of open systems and distributed systems are enabling organizations to make the transition from maintaining older legacy systems toward taking an enterprise network approach to systems development.

**List serve**   A specific list server, which is any program that distributes messages to a mailing list on the Internet.

**Load**   To enter a program into the computer from cartridge, cassette, disk, or CD.

**Local area network (LAN)**   A system of network software and hardware components used to connect a group of end stations by means of a wire cable or fiber-optic link. A single LAN segment connects from one to several hundred end stations, usually in the same building. A large organization may have as many as 1,000 or more LAN segments and tens of thousands of end stations.

**Log-on**   A sign-in procedure.

**Longitudinal patient record**   A record, either electronic or on paper, outlining a patient's lifetime medical history, showing diagnoses, treatments, pharmacological interventions, and other health care efforts.

**Lycos**   A web "spider" that helps users locate resources using keyword searches.

**M**   A computer programming language originated at Massachusetts General Hospital in the late 1960s and 1970s. Formerly known as MUMPS, an acronym for the Massachusetts General Hospital Utility Multiprogramming System, is now used in many different industries in addition to health care.

**Machine readable**   The ability to use specialized equipment to read data from a source and create electronic transactions for processing or data file access.

**Magnetic stripe**   A plastic card technology, applied to credit cards and health care identification cards, that uses a magnetic surface encoded with data supporting read-only functionality in conformance with standards from the American National Standards Institute.

**Magnetic tape**   Flexible plastic tape, on one side of which is a uniform coating of dispersed magnetic material, in which signals are registered for subsequent reproduction. Used for registering television images, sound, or computer data.

**Mailing list**   A list of e-mail addresses to which messages, usually on a specific topic, are sent.

**Mainframe**   A large, fast, and powerful computer with enormous disk capacity designed to process large amounts of data and to serve a very high number of users using different applications at the same time.

**Management services organization (MSO)**   A legal entity that provides practice management services to a hospital, physicians, or a physician-hospital organization. The MSO may own the facilities and employ the nonphysician staff used to deliver care.

**Master patient index (MPI)**   A relational database application that lists all the identification numbers assigned to one patient in all the information systems in a hospital or integrated delivery system. It then assigns a global identification number for each patient, which is used in the background to locate a patient's medical records in an enterprisewide system.

**Medical information system (MIS)**   A term used interchangeably with HIS.

**Megabyte (MB)**   1 million bytes or 8 million bits.

**Memory**   The internal part of a computer (found in the CPU) where programs and data are stored.

**Memory card**   Using a memory computer chip that is not as sophisticated as a microprocessor chip, the card can contain as many as 256 characters. Such cards are used in other countries to identify patients.

**Microcomputer**   A small desktop computer.

**Microprocessor**   Another name for the CPU chip.

**Midrange**   A computer platform or system that typically has less processing power than mainframe systems, but more power than workstations or microcomputers. A midrange is sometimes referred to as a minicomputer.

**Minicomputer**   A larger and more powerful computer than a microcomputer.

**Mirroring**   A data protection method in which a backup storage device maintains data identical to that on the primary device, thus serving as a backup in case the primary unit fails.

**Mission critical**   Information tied to top-priority business processes.

**Modem**   Modulator/Demodulator. A device used to change computer codes into pulses or signals that can travel over telephone lines.

**Monitor**   Video device; quality of display is better than that of a television set.

**Multimedia**   Hardware and software that is capable of delivering not only text but also digitized voice, image, and/or video presentations of information.

**Multiplexer**   The traditional device for dividing a long-distance, high-speed telecommunications line so that it can be shared by many users. Used extensively in wide area networks, it provides for the concurrent transmission of multiple information signals on a single data channel by apportioning the time available on the composite channel for individual signals or by assigning specific frequencies for each information signal. High-end routers can interface directly with wide area communication services, reducing the need for multiplexers.

**Multipurpose Internet mail extension (MIME)**   The standard for attaching nontext files, such as graphics, spreadsheets, formatted work processing files, and others, to standard Internet messages.

**Narrowband network**   A network that carries significantly less information, no more than 64,000 bits of information per second, than a broadband network. It is used for traditional telephone service, electronic mail, paging services, and facsimile transmission.

**National information infrastructure**   An interconnected communications network consisting of computers and workstations, software applications and databases, and technical standards for linking users.

**Network**   A collection of hardware, such as printers, modems, servers, and clients, that enables users to store and retrieve information, share devices, and exchange information.

**Neural network**   In sharp contrast to an expert system, a neural network is a highly mathematical learning methodology that learns from many examples to properly categorize new examples. Neural networks were inspired by the interconnectivity of neurons in the human brain, and they have tremendous ability to perform pattern recognition.

**Newsgroup**   A discussion group on a specific topic, maintained on a computer network or a bulletin board.

**Node**   A station on a network that can communicate with other such stations.

**Nomenclature and vocabulary**   A consistent method of assigning names to elements of a system.

**Nursing informatics**   The discipline of applying computer science to nursing processes.

**Nursing minimum data set (NMDS)**   An essential set of information that has uniform definitions and categories concerned with nursing functions.

**Object linking and embedding (OLE)**   A Microsoft Corporation protocol for application-to-application exchange and communication using data objects. Date objects can be either embedded or linked. OLE for Health Care is designed specifically for use in linking health care front-end applications.

**Object-oriented database**   A database organized around an object model, rather than the more conventional relational or flat models. This type of database allows for grouping of many different types and sources of data. It provides a data model that is closer to the way humans think about data than is the relational database.

**Object-oriented technology**   A computer programming approach that builds software applications through the repeated use of self-contained object-bits of data that are surrounded with the program information. Objects can perform certain computer functions when they receive messages to do that function.

**Off-line**   Not installed in or connected to the computer. Tapes and disks that have been unmounted from the computer are off-line. Terminals, printers, or any other devices that are turned off, though still physically connected to the computer, are considered off-line.

**On-line** Pertaining to equipment or software that is directly connected to and performing operations on the CPU.

**On-line, real-time EDI** Providing an immediate response to a computerized request, such as a health insurance eligibility inquiry. Unlike interactive EDI, on-line, real-time systems do not permit instantaneous follow-up communications.

**On-line terminal** The operation of terminals, disks, and other equipment under direct and absolute control of the central processor to eliminate the need for human intervention at any stage between initial input and computer output.

**Open systems** Systems based on technology and protocols that can be employed by multiple vendors. Standards-based open systems are based on publicly accepted conventions that are available to all vendors. Open systems, in theory, can operate with any system that follows those conventions.

**Operating system (OS)** The set of computer programs that controls the inner workings of the computer. It ties together the various peripherals and the other hardware components of the computer system, and it manages tasks requested by the application programs.

**Optical card** Using the same technology as a compact disk, the card can contain as many as 4 million characters of memory that can be updated. The card is in the conceptual stage for health care applicants.

**Optical character recognition (OCR)** An imaging technology that uses a scanning device to convert paper documents to electronic alphanumeric characters that can be stored on a computer.

**Outcomes research** Studies that assess the end results of medical treatment, generally measured in terms of a patient's ability to function, quality of life, and length of life.

**Output** Information transferred from internal storage to an output device.

**Output device** A device or machine that delivers information for the computer to the operator.

**Packet** A collection of bits that includes data and other control information, such as source and destination addresses for nodes on a network.

**Packet filter** The ability to select a route for a packet based on a prescribed set of criteria, such as its source, destination, or length, thus facilitating network traffic.

**Parallel interface** A port that sends or receives the eight bits, in each byte, all at one time. Many printers likely to be used in the home use a parallel interface to connect to the computer.

**Patient accounting system** A software program, typically used in providers' business offices, that posts charges for services delivered to patients, sends bills, and keeps track of amounts owed and how long bills are outstanding.

**PC-DOS** IBM's name for the disk operating system used in the IBM personal computer.

**Peripherals** Accessory parts of a computer system that are not considered essential to its operation. Printers and modems are peripherals.

**Picture archiving and communications system (PACS)** A database system in which one or more radiologic modalities—X-ray, ultrasound, or computed tomagraphy, for example—are stored and distributed by a network image server to workstations. The system typically allows manipulation and comparisons of images.

**Point-of-sale (POS) device** A manually operated reader with a long, narrow channel or slot through which the edge of a credit card or ID card is pushed, thereby moving the machine readable portion of the card past a reading station.

**Port** The point at which a communication network terminates at a network, series, or parallel interface card.

**Practice guidelines** Recommendations, developed by private or public organizations, regarding the most appropriate diagnostic and treatment approaches for an individual with a particular medical problem. Also known as critical pathways or treatment protocols.

**Practitioner** Any individual who provides health care to patients, including physicians, nurses, and therapists.

**Printer** Transforms computer output into hard copy.

**Process management** Assuring the organization that each process meets quality, cost, and productivity improvement standards or goals. Processes can be defined, measured, and systematically proven.

**Program** Shortened form of "computer program." A set of stored instructions in a computer that direct the actions within the computer.

**Programmable read-only memory (PROM)** A type of ROM that can be changed, but only with a high degree of expertise.

**Protocol** Computer end stations each have their own set of conventions or protocols that they use to format data and establish connections across a network. Unix devices employ transmission control protocol/Internet protocol (TCP/IP); Digital Electronic Corporation computers use the DECnet protocol; IBM mainframes traditionally communicate with systems network architecture (SNA); Novell servers use the Netware IPX protocol. A high-end, multiprotocol router can accommodate all major local area network/wide area network protocols on the same physical internetwork.

**Provider** Any type of individual or organization that provides patient care, including physicians, nurses, therapists, hospitals, health maintenance organizations, clinics, and so on.

**Provider profiling** The collection and analysis of claims and benefits management data for the identification of cost, utilization, and quality of care characteristics of physicians, health care facilities, and allied health providers.

**Random access memory (RAM)**   Also known as read-write memory, this part of internal memory is known as temporary memory.

**Read**   To extract data from a computer's memory or from a tape or disk.

**Reader**   The electromechanical device used to extract data from previously encoded media, such as a magnetic stripe card.

**Read-only memory (ROM)**   A kind of internal memory that cannot be changed.

**Real-time**   A description of an action or system capable of computing at a speed commensurate with the time of occurrence of an actual process.

**Redundant array of inexpensive disk (RAID)**   A method of storing data on multiple hard disk drives for faster access and/or greater reliability. There are six officially defined levels, each designed for a specific kind of application.

**Reference database**   A public or private database containing aggregate data about many patients or cases that can be used for effectiveness research, financial analyses, and other purposes.

**Relational database**   A database model in which information is stored in two-dimensional tables, consisting of rows and columns. The rows represent records, and the columns represent data fields, which are the pieces that form the entry record. Relational databases allow easy comparison of data, and multiple entries can be updated in separate databases through a change in one database.

**Reliability, availability, serviceability (RAS)**   Key measurements of a network's life cycle costs.

**Remittance advice**   A statement sent to providers that outlines how a payer adjudicated a claim and paid for services. A payer may also send a remittance statement summarizing all remittance advice for a particular payment period.

**Remote computing**   A form of outsourcing where a client's personal computers are networked into a vendor's data processing center via high-speed phone lines. Rapid response times allow the client to access software at the vendor's site as if it were down the hall. Thus, a client avoids hardware costs and shares processing and software costs with the vendor's other remote processing clients.

**Reset**   To reset the computer and its peripherals to a starting state before beginning a task. Done automatically by the disk operating system.

**Ring network**   A network topology in the form of a closed loop or circle, with each node in the network connected to each other. Messages move in one direction around the system. When a message arrives at a node, the node examines the address information in the message. If the address matches the node's address, the message is accepted. Otherwise, the node regenerates the signal and places it back on the network. Ring networks normally use some form of token-passing protocol to regulate network traffic.

**Robotics** A general term used for industrial robots that are used to increase production. An example is the use of computer-controlled robots in automobile assembly lines.

**Router** The primary interconnecting device, a router is an intelligent, high-performance means of connecting local area networks or wide area networks. Unlike bridges, routers maintain an internal representation or topology of the physical links in a network. With their knowledge of the Internet work topology, routers can send data traffic among end stations efficiently, quickly, and reliably.

**Scroll** To move a video display up or down, line by line, or side to side, character by character.

**Search engines** Software that uses queries to find information on the Internet or an intranet. Search engines look on Web servers, either through a directory of Web sites or through Web pages themselves, to find information that matches a user's query. Several search engines can be accessed directly on the Internet by typing in an Internet address.

**Seat** A workstation connected to an asynchronous transfer mode switch or other kind of network.

**Segmentation** Improving a network's performance by dividing a large network into several smaller, less congested local area networks, while maintaining connectivity between them. This is efficiently done through the use of switches, which further aid the process of facilitating network traffic because they can carry many transmissions simultaneously.

**Self-funding** A method of financing health coverage in which employers fund benefit plans from their own resources without purchasing insurance. Such plans may be self-administered, or the employer may contract with a third-party administrator or an insurance company for administrative services only.

**Server** The system hardware that provides services, such as information or computer programs, to the client in the client-server system.

**Service bureau** An organization that offers data processing of claims and time-sharing services for hospitals and physicians. These outsourcing arrangements often include accounts receivable services and other benefits. Access to these organizations is gained either through leased or private lines or packet switching networks.

**Simple network management protocol (SNMP)** The protocol under the transmission control protocol/Internet protocol suite for network management. SNMP provides a means to monitor and set network configurations and other variables.

**Software** The general term for sets of computer instructions (programs) that manage the general facilities of the computer and control the operation of application programs.

**Source code**   The software code that is written by a programmer. The code is converted by a compiler into a form that is meaningful to the computer processing hardware.

**Standard prescriber identification number**   Under development by the National Council of Prescription Drug Programs in conjunction with other professional organizations, this standard number could be used to identify prescribers.

**Standard query language (SQL)**   A standardized database search language that enables quick searches of vast amounts of information in either one relational database or across several relational databases. SQL is used to both define and access the information in such databases.

**Standards**   Clearly defined and agreed-upon conventions for the operation and behavior of specific computing functions, formats, and processes. Open standards are those that are developed through a process in which all interested parties can participate.

**Star network**   A network topology in the form of a star. At the center of the star is a wiring hub or concentrator, and the nodes or workstations are arranged around the central point.

**Storage**   Usually refers to long-term storage.

**Store and forward operation**   A data transmission model that uses a form of message switching that temporarily stores messages in intermediate points before sending them to their next destinations.

**Structured text**   Concepts and ideas that are described in text but are assigned codes so that they can be recognized and analyzed by a computer.

**Support**   Help available from computer and software vendors.

**Switch**   A device with several ports that can support one workstation or an entire local area network. It works quickly to move packets between local area networks attached to each port.

**Switch Digital Service-56**   High-speed transmission technology that transmits data at 56,000 bits per second and is used for videoconferencing and telecommuting applications.

**Switched multimegabit data service (SMDS)**   A high-speed, fast packet service that transmits data in packets, or electronic envelopes, at rates ranging from 1.5 million to 45 million bits per second. SMDS is best suited for high-volume data applications, such as interconnecting data networks or linking mainframe computers.

**Symbolic reasoning**   A method of deduction that follows an explicit line of inferences. In contrast to traditional computer programming languages, artificial intelligence programs using symbolic reasoning enable more complex reasoning.

**System**   A group of actions or procedures that are logically connected by their operation and products and that together accomplish a connected set of organizational objectives.

**Systematized Nomenclature of Human and Veterinary Medicine (Snomed)**   A standardized vocabulary belonging to the College of American Pathologist, Northfield,

IL. Many experts consider Snomed to be the best starting point for developing a standardized vocabulary for computer-based patient records.

**Taxonomy**   A method of classifying a vocabulary of terms for a specific topic according to specific laws or principles.

**Telecommunications infrastructure**   The underlying structure or framework of the telecommunication system; the cable, conduit, switching machines, amplifiers, and support systems that permit the transmission of voice, video, and data.

**Telecommuting**   Working at home with a terminal.

**Terabyte (TB)**   In computing, 1 trillion bytes, or 1 million megabytes. Terabytes are used to represent extremely large memory capacities.

**Terminal**   A device used to transmit and receive data over communication lines to and from the computer.

**Third-party administrator**   An administrative organization used by a self-funded employer to collect premiums, pay claims, and/or provide administrative services.

**Three-tier architecture**   A client-server system in which the central host or mainframe, desktop client systems, and intermediate servers all work cooperatively in a coordinated three-level, client-server computing approach.

**Token ring network**   This network structure uses a circulating electronic token to prevent several nodes from transmitting on the network simultaneously.

**T1**   A long-distance, point-to-point circuit providing 24 channels of 64 kilobits per second, for a total of 1.544 megabits per second. It is a building block of digital communications service from a common carrier for voice or data transmission.

**Topology**   The "map" of a network. In physical terms, it may refer to where cables are run and where other devices, such as nodes, gateways, routers, and servers, are located.

**Translation software**   Programs that convert an organization's business application formats to a standard format, and vice versa, when information is electronically transmitted between trading partners.

**Transmission control protocol/Internet protocol (TCP/IP)**   A set of communication protocols encompassing media access, packet transport, session communications, file transfer, electronic mail, and terminal emulation. It is supported by a large number of hardware and software vendors, and it is also the basis of the Internet. TCP conducts data transfer between computers on the Internet or an intranet, and it ensures data is transmitted correctly. IP takes data from the TCP, breaks the data into packets, and ships the data to another network.

**Turnkey**   A term used to describe a hardware-software combination that comes in a "package." There are no changes or options; the package must run the way it is.

**Universal resource locator (URL)**   A string of characters that identifies the location of a document of the World Wide Web.

**Unix**   A computer operating system originally developed by AT&T and now widely available in a number of different variations.

**Usenet**   A large group of networks and computers that organizes messages by newsgroup; a branch of the Internet.

**Valid value**   All of the possible data elements that could be assigned to a particular category of information. For example, if the category is "month," the valid values would be January, February, and so on.

**Value-added network (VAN)**   The vehicle for carrying data from the point of service to the point of receipt, including both the network and switch functions. In health care, VANs can serve as the vehicle for transmitting claims, supply orders, and other transactions.

**Veronica**   A frequently updated index system intended to make gopher an even easier tool to use.

**Voice recognition**   Systems that enable physicians, nurses, and other caregivers to enter information in patients' charts simply by talking to a computer, eliminating the need for dictation devices, keyboards, light pens, mouses, and other means of data entry. Approaches involve template matching, which works by matching acoustical images of spoken words with a database, and continuous speech recognition, which has a larger database vocabulary and can understand works in context.

**Web server**   A networked computer that stores and transmits documents written in hypertext markup language, the formatting language for Web-based documents, and other data to browsers via the hypertext transport protocol, an Internet-based data transfer protocol.

**Wide area information server (WAIS)**   An automated Internet search that allows users to locate documents containing key words or phrases.

**Wide area network (WAN)**   A collection of long-distance telecommunication links and networks used to connect local area networks and end stations across regional, national, or international distances.

**Wideband network**   A network that carries less information—between 64,000 and 1.5 million bits of information per second—than a broadband network, but more than a narrowband network. It is used for video teleconferencing and file transfer.

**Work flow systems**   The automation or streamlining of processes. Work flow systems usually are based on electronic versions of documents and how they are routed through departments in a company, which transactions have to be accomplished in which order, and what to do about exceptions and mistakes.

**World Wide Web**   A hypertext data framework that operates on the Internet. The Web has home pages with links to other pages. These can be graphica. with "buttons" for jumping to most locations anywhere on the Web. Most Web browsing programs, such as Mosaic and Netscape, maintain a list of places visited in a single session and allow a user to bookmark places so they can be revisited easily.

**Write**  To enter information into memory or onto a tape or disk.

# INDEX